SOCIAL INFORMATION SCIENCE

To Eric
with love

SOCIAL INFORMATION SCIENCE

Love, Health and the Information Society

Shifra Baruchson-Arbib

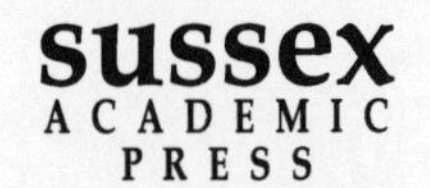

Published 1996 by
SUSSEX ACADEMIC PRESS
18 Chichester Place
Brighton BN2 1FF, United Kingdom

Distributed in the United States by
International Specialized Book Services, Inc.
5804 N.E. Hassalo St.
Portland, Oregon 97213–3644
USA

British Library Cataloguing in Publication Data
A CIP catalogue record for this book is available from the British Library.

ISBN 1–898723 36 2

Copy-edited and typeset in 10 on 12½ Sabon and Helvetica
by Grahame & Grahame Editorial, Brighton, East Sussex
Printed and bound by Biddles Ltd, King's Lynn and Guildford

Contents

Preface and Acknowledgments

A research study I conducted on reading habits and literacy in Renaissance Italy was the beginning of a fascinating journey that taught me about the love, spirit, and collective wisdom found in books. Leaving behind the magnificent world of ancient manuscripts and rare books, I entered the world of the future as head of the Department of Information Studies and Librarianship at Bar-Ilan University, Israel. But I could not leave the past behind completely, and while developing the department toward future technology I questioned myself as to whether the love and comfort that are found in books would disappear as the information revolution, and its technological repercussions, begins to shape our lives. Surely there had to be a means whereby the new technology could serve as an agent to better the lives of all.

With these thoughts in mind, I embarked on a new journey, no less fascinating than the first one, to find out what are the basic human needs that can be fulfilled through books, information, and high-tech technology. I learned that in the unstable and high-pressure world we live in, men and women need an anchor to hold on to in times of crisis, social distress, and health problems. This anchor may be found by acquiring the right information at the right time, by finding a variety of alternative solutions in times of crises and problems, and, above all, by finding a source of aid, support, and encouragement. I discovered that all these needs could be fulfilled either completely or partially with the help of books and information. These sources of strength are known to western society, but it is necessary to find new methods in order to make them available for millions of people in an easy, uncomplicated way. What is needed is a merger between people's basic needs and the new opportunities that the information revolution offers us.

The way forward presented here is to form a new academic discipline – "Social Information Science" (SI Science). Development of this new branch of study would expose us to new social and technological concepts, to new social establishments, and to the new profession of "Social Information Scientist." SI Science may become the new science of the 21st century. It has the power to help turn our society into a unique "Information Society," a society with soul, love, and well-being.

While conducting this research, I met and was assisted by many interesting and loving people who encouraged me to write this book: Ms R. Brown, the bibliotherapist at St. Elizabeth's Hospital in Washington, D.C.; the late Dr E. Mundt and Dr C. Adeney of "The Happy Children's Ward" at the University Hospital in Munich; S. Goldstone of the New York Training Institute for Neurolinguistic Programming; Ms D. Goldschmidt, the information scientist at Bar-Ilan University; and Ms S. Victor, who assisted with the English translation.

I would like to take this opportunity to thank the Rector of Bar-Ilan University, Prof. M. Kaveh, and Vice-President for Research, Prof. S. Grossman, for their support in carrying out the research.

This book is dedicated to my husband, Eric, whose constant love and support encouraged me to complete this book.

Dr Shifra Baruchson-Arbib
July 1995
Bar-Ilan University, Israel

The paper world we lived in for so long may and perhaps should be supplanted by an electronic counterpart. But in this transformation we have a chance to improve the world – a one-time chance.

T. H. Nelson

1

Technology and Humanitarianism at the Crossroads

As we approach the millennium, at the gates of the 21st century, we are on the way to a "paperless society,"[1] a society with a wealth of technological and computerized means. Along with the removal of barriers between the various sciences, and the development of interdisciplinary fields of research, the methods for location and distribution of information have become easier and quicker. The last quarter of the 20th century has been characterized by the invention of sophisticated computers, data bases, complex communication networks such as the Internet and Bitnet, electronic mail, sophisticated software, artificial intelligence, expert systems, electronic books, and talking books. All of these, and, certainly, other future inventions, will transform the society in which we live into something different, a society characterized by swift means of communication and modernized methods of reading, studying, locating, and processing information.[2]

It is impossible to predict what the social and psychological effects of these phenomena will be. It is clear that our methods of information acquisition will change. It is possible, though not certain, that the object we know as a book will gradually become rare, just as the manuscript form disappeared after Gutenberg's invention of the printing press in 1440; and then again, maybe not. It is conceivable that the information technologies will be used mainly for research and data retrieval, while the book will be preserved and will continue to be read for leisure entertainment and enjoyment. It is quite feasible that 21st-century man may not want to give up the exclusive, individual and emotional experience associated with reading literary works and poetry, whereas the individual requiring factual data in the fields of research, commerce, or industry, will be able to obtain this information in a rapid, computerized way, without the necessity of tediously browsing through books. We are already in the process of an information revolution: the world is turning into one huge library without walls. An example of one such giant library can already be seen in the "Gutenberg Project," established in 1971 at Illinois Benedictine College, in the United States. This project, headed by Professor Michael Hart, has an ambitious goal: the free distribution of a trillion "electronic texts" by the end of the year 2001.[3]

The specialization of location and organization of information will become an essential profession in the new era. The Information scientist will be acquainted with the newly-developing technologies and will have the unique professional expertise needed to process, categorize, organize, and distribute information. Alongside these tremendous ongoing technological developments, problems are certain to arise in areas such as securing information, copyright, the protection of privacy, respect for the public's right to know, and coping with the new computer addiction – Computer Mania.[4]

At a time when many are becoming aware of this new revolution and are engrossed in familiarizing themselves with new technologies, this book examines the use of human knowledge from a different angle: one that bridges the gap between the ancient and the new – linking humanitarianism with modern techniques, delineating the soul of writers with the needs of man. The purpose of this book is to find a point of contact between the needs of society, human knowledge, and technological developments. The heritage of knowledge is examined from a new point of view – as a unique source for helping people, a source of aid, welfare, and support. I propose the establishment of a new academic discipline, "Social Information Science" (SI Science), which will help meet the social needs of modern man by webbing the written heritage of humanity with modern technology. The idea that inspired this book was the recognition of the basic difference between the printing revolution of the 15th century and the information revolution of our times. The importance of the printing press was enormous, but it happened accidentally; it was not planned. Even Gutenberg himself, while printing the 42-line Bible using a huge format and letter style similar to old manuscripts, had no idea of the future economic and literary potential of the printed book. But now, approaching the 21st century, after a century which has witnessed the development of the social sciences, and knowing the potential effect of technological inventions, it is possible to plan at least part of the future and guide the new technologies in a positive and productive direction.[5]

By nature, every invention can be used either constructively or destructively. From the inventor and modern researcher, we expect not only excellence in the field of research, but also high moral values. Some of the major inventions of the 20th century, such as nuclear arms and genetic science, can be used either to build or to destroy. Even in the advanced world of information, modern technology can be used in a constructive or a destructive way. The new information technology can be used to make advances in science and to make life easier for mankind. However, it can also be used to destroy: sophisticated computer software can violate an individual's privacy, distort data, mislead, and produce information specifically for the purpose of gaining control and making a profit. It is even possible that the cultural treasures of human history will lose their reading audience in the wake of the enthusiasm over technological progress.[6] George Orwell's *Nineteen Eighty-four* could well come true in the 21st century. Without open and thorough discussions between specialists in the humanities, the social science fields, and computer experts, a situation could be reached where we find ourselves in a society that has no room for individuality, where power is in the hands of those tangled in webs of information and communication secrets. Man is free to choose between good and evil, destruction and construction. With a responsible attitude, and by acting in a cautious manner, man can transform the new information technologies into a positive power that can bring enlightenment to our universe.

The need for awareness of the importance of information in the new world is clearly understood by politicians. In a speech given by President Bill Clinton at the American University in Washington on February 26, 1992, he presented a program for action, and listed US priorities in the framework of international economics. In his speech, the President referred to the importance of information and its role in his program. Among other things, he said: "But the most important thing [i.e. information] is that information has become global and has been crowned king of world economics. In the past, wealth was measured by land, gold, oil, and cars; today the main indicator of our wealth is information, its quality, quantity and the speed in which it can be obtained. The value and quantity of information have soared to new heights."

A few days earlier, President Clinton had revealed the principles of his technological policy in a 36-page report presented to the public. According to this policy document, over the next four years 17 billion dollars would be invested in the encouragement of cooperation between the private sector and the Administration for the promotion of advanced technological projects. Included in the framework of the five-part program presented in the report was a project to establish a nationwide communications network – the "Information Superhighway" – a network that would be capable of transferring data in high-level files. The main goal of this project, which was inspired and supported by the enthusiasm and good will of Vice President Al Gore, is to create nationwide networking for US residents, institutions, and official and private information suppliers. This network, which is based on optic fiber, is expected to open a new world of possibilities to the public for obtaining information from any source, on any topic and for any purpose. Mark Cooper, research director of CFA (Consumerism Federation of America), claims that the acquisition of this network will open new markets and unlimited business opportunities to the high-tech industries. Experts predict that such a "highway" network will accelerate the transition of white-collar workers to

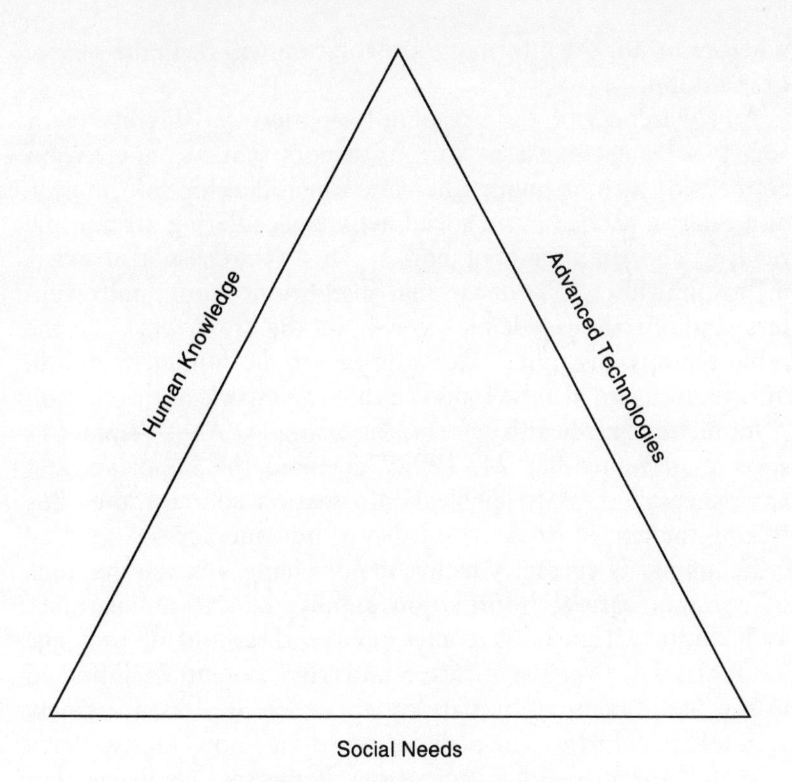

The Triangle of Social Information Science

"work at home," and, in addition, the project will provide new opportunities for computer programmers and scientists leaving the defense industry.[7]

There is no doubt that the Clinton Program will bring about a tremendous transformation in the possible methods of acquiring, transferring, buying, and selling information. The program is technical in character, and will lead us to a "new information age." However, along with the technical possibilities opening up to us, the question still to be asked is whether the new information age will merely be a symbol for genius technology or, perhaps, alongside the information revolution, a new humanitarian revolution will develop that can make use of the new communications systems for the benefit and support of the human race. The true question is whether or not the information revolution will be in the service of mankind.

An awareness of the use of information and literature for society's benefit exists in various sectors that are not always connected, such as public libraries, which develop information and referral services, and social activities centering around the reading and discussing of books. This awareness also exists in hospital libraries, educational institutions, community centers and, in the academic world, in the framework of the bibliotherapy discipline. Recognition of the human factor in information can also be found in the framework of the Clinton Administration's health reform; for example, in the President's speech on September 24, 1992, he noted the importance of having easy access to medical information sources, and thus freeing the citizen from the burden of bureaucracy.[8]

Humanity is currently facing major changes in the methods of communication, information supply, education, learning, and reading. This book comes on the threshold of that age – to cast light on the positive and vital potential embodied in the old systems of human knowledge as well as in its new technological forms. The positive use of the knowledge we have inherited from previous generations is the real challenge that will face humankind in the 21st century.

2

Human Knowledge as a Source of Aid and Support

Information and Literary Works

Human knowledge is the product of thousands of years of collective thought and effort. In effect, what we have is an international library which houses global knowledge in a variety of forms: books, articles, newspapers, video–audio cassettes, CD-Rom, and data bases. This vast quantity of knowledge has been handed down to us throughout history in a variety of forms: factual and numerical data, scientific research, commentaries, reviews, as well as belles-lettres, poetry, and drama. If we attempt to visualize this great international library, we can see a huge accumulation of information from all periods of human existence, information which is amazing, fascinating, and irreplaceable.

We tend to divide human knowledge into two key categories: direct information and literature. Under the information category is the vast storehouse of knowledge which includes numerical data, factual data (such as names, addresses, institutions, and organizations), and more complex data such as scientific research, reviews, critiques, commentaries, newspapers, and legal books. This knowledge is necessary for our day-to-day existence, and for the development of the various research branches. The second category, the field of literature, is composed of poetry, prose, and plays: compositions of creative and spiritual substance which enrich our lives and provide enjoyment and entertainment. This vast wealth of knowledge can be divided further by using the traditional systems of classification. Seeing things from the broadest perspective, it seems that people approach human knowledge from two main viewpoints, the practical and the spiritual. The first helps people cope in everyday life, and the second supplies recreation and nourishment for the soul.

Nowadays, when we mention the terms "human knowledge" and "information" we subconsciously visualize computers, data bases, and CD-Roms. But if we could just put aside for a moment the conservative, conventional approach, we would find – in addition to electronic means, information, and literature – a "treasure," an amazing source of aid, assistance, and support for the human race. Among the practical and literary knowledge, we would find unique tools stemming from the conscious and unconscious human experience and emotions. Discovering these tools and developing innovative methods for their use in conjunction with the new technological means would bring humanity a step forward.

Aid and Support

In order to function as a healthy, active, and stable society, mankind needs the right information at the right time, as well as emotional encouragement and support. During the 20th century, attempts were made to organize human information in a systematic and easy-to-use way. The professions of librarianship and information science were conceived to enable ordinary people to find their way easily around the complicated global library. In this book I suggest that we take a short break from the technological rat-race, that we turn off the computers for a while, close the Dewey classification books, and look in a new way at the huge accumulation of human knowledge which includes information, experience, and emotions. This short break is imperative for any attempt to answer the inevitable question: how can this knowledge be used for the benefit of people and society? Before we try to answer this, it is important to explain that, in using the terms "aid," "support," and "relief," the broadest possible definition is intended. Any direct or indirect information or knowledge that might be useful for someone in temporary or permanent distress can be defined as a source of aid. This means that any knowledge that is used to help, to find a solution or an alternative, or even just some simple relief, is important as a tool for helping people. In other words, any possible knowledge – from simple information, such as the name of an institution or organization, to the information concealed in belles-lettres, which may provide the reader with a figure to identify with, a novel solution, or a fresh insight – is a source of help and support. I refer here not only to the information found in the printed book, but also to the vast knowledge found in advanced technological forms: data bases, electronic mail (E-mail), electronic publishing, the talking book, and multimedia systems, which could all be applied in original ways to benefit and help the public.[1]

The Consumer: People in Need

Human knowledge (composed of information, literature, and technology) and aid, support, and relief (in all possible shapes and forms), needs to be matched to the needs of the consumer. Just as the first two components are described here in the broadest sense, so too the "public" means all human beings who need advice, the right information at the right time, comfort, support, and encouragement. Most people need assistance at certain times during their lives: for example, parents coping with education and health issues; children and teens coping with personal relationships; and people in times of emotional stress – family crises (divorce and death), transitional periods (growing up and growing old), and social and health problems. People in trouble require basic information and support in order to be able to deal with their problems.[2] The help received through information and literary knowledge is not a miracle cure, but it does lead to a positive and creative approach, openness and understanding (through exposure to a selection of possible solutions), and encouragement and relief through

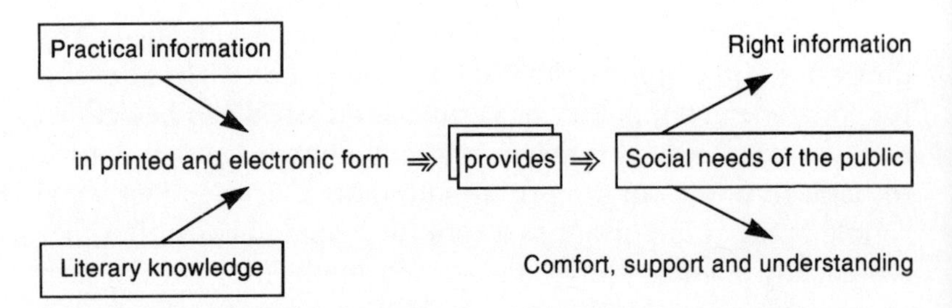

A New Overview of Human Knowledge and its Utilization

identification with similar situations. Having the appropriate information at the right time enables people in distress to feel that they are in control, that they at least have the basic tools to cope with their situation. (I am not referring here to people in mental or physical distress, who need specialized help, but to the general population with everyday problems.)

Here are a few examples where relevant information can help. Let us begin with something very basic: children of old or sick parents, speculating on the best institution for their parents. It is important for them to know if there are any voluntary support organizations, and what their social rights are as regards receiving financial help. Divorced parents needing up-to-date information on the right psychological approach to take with their children might find just the right book, and maybe even locate support groups. As another example: the parents of a child with a chronic disease, or – conversely – children of seriously ill parents with diseases like cancer, Alzheimer's, Aids, etc., desperately need basic information about the disease, its side effects, and possibilities for medical and social assistance. Any basic information, such as names of institutions, and new or alternative treatments, is of enormous help. A book or film dealing with a person in identical circumstances may enable these people to look at their own situations from a different viewpoint and, perhaps, to find tools for coping. A patient in a rehabilitation institution, a wounded soldier or an accident victim, may well find comfort in the biography of a person who experienced similar difficulties and finally succeeded in overcoming them. A perfect example is President Franklin D.

Roosevelt, who was paralyzed in both legs, yet still succeeded in becoming one of the most prominent presidents of the United States. A disabled person who cannot hold a book may find some relief by using a "talking book." There are numerous and varied examples, and the subject of aid through information is a topic worthy of another book.

Many societies throughout the world are enlightened; people are interested in information concerning their lives. The development of fields such as "patient education" and "preventive medicine," especially in the United States and Great Britain, is an indication of the growing need for information. As R. Gann writes in his study on health and information: "People are no longer content to be told what is good for them: they want access to information which will enable them to weigh up risks and benefits and to make informed choices between options in health care."[3]

The need for appropriate medical information – on institutions, treatment methods, new technologies, aid organizations – will, no doubt, become an integral part of life in the 21st century. The public will be exposed to both new and old methods of aid and treatment, and will need background information in order to find the most suitable solutions. When we travel abroad, we go first to a travel agent, select the appropriate tour, compare prices, examine the services offered by the travel agency, and only then do we make our decision. When we buy an apartment, we go to a real estate agent or read the ads in the newspaper, examine alternatives, look at apartments, and compare prices. When we buy a dress we often go window shopping first; however, when we are faced with social or health problems we are initially confused. Some seek an appropriate solution and find one, while others engage in exhausting efforts to find a solution and may even reach the conclusion that there is none. Appropriate information given at the right time with a kind word is a primary tool in relieving distress. Just as the traffic light directs traffic and prevents accidents, so the right information and sources of support at the right time can lead to a positive and constructive course of action.

3

"Mrs Jones" in 1995 and 2025

In order to demonstrate the importance of receiving appropriate information and support at the right time, I will present an imaginary case – the case of Mrs Jones. We will accompany Mrs Jones through one year of her life – 1995 – and then describe the same, imaginary case 30 years later, in the year 2025. The case will be identical, but will the results be the same?

Mrs Jones is a middle-class high-school teacher living in Connecticut, USA. She is married to Mark Jones, a building engineer; the couple have two children, a six-year-old boy and a fifteen-year-old girl. The couple's relationship has begun to deteriorate and, after years of conflict, they obtain a divorce in 1995, with the mother retaining custody of the children. Mrs Jones now begins a new life as a single mother. She must support the family, educate the children and also cope with an elderly mother who lives close by. We will observe Mrs Jones during the first year after her divorce and see how she manages.

Immediately after the divorce, Mrs Jones is in a poor emotional state. The only person giving her support is her neighbor, Jill, who is a good friend. When Mrs Jones's six-year-old son, Jimmy, starts school he has trouble adjusting, lacks patience, and is unable to make new friends. Mrs Jones quickly turns to the school's guidance counselor, who refers her to the psychological counseling services. The child refuses to attend the sessions with the psychologist. The mother, who had expected Jimmy to excel in school like his older sister, Anne, is frustrated. The atmosphere at home is charged and tense. Toward the end of the year, and as a result of a conversation with her friend

Jill, Mrs Jones begins to suspect that her son's problem is not one of laziness, but, rather, an organic problem – dyslexia. A well-known physician confirms that the child is indeed dyslexic. The mother, who is under-informed on the subject, is horrified and consumed by guilt. The boy soon begins undergoing treatment with a psychologist, and the pressure at home is somewhat alleviated as he slowly begins accepting his disability and learns to deal with it.

At about the same time, Mrs Jones's mother suffers a stroke. She remains lucid, but becomes paralyzed, and in need of constant care. Mrs Jones is tense and nervous; her life seems to be falling apart. Her mother requires around-the-clock nursing and attention; she must locate a wheelchair for her, and rearrange her mother's room to suit her changed physical abilities. Mrs Jones is constantly criticized by her mother, and this reactivates her feelings of guilt. Her financial situation worsens so that she cannot afford to hire private help for her mother, yet her feelings of guilt prevent her from committing her to a hospital or nursing home. After months of devoted care, a now despondent Mrs Jones begins finding out about nursing homes for her mother. Most of them are very expensive, and the pressures mount. In the meantime, her fifteen-year-old daughter Anne, a previously brilliant student of above average intelligence, is showing the strain of her parents' divorce; she is torn between her love for her father and for her mother, and is unable to cope with seeing her mother's worsening mental condition. The girl has trouble finding her niche at school and begins to regress. One day her mother catches her taking drugs. Mrs Jones collapses and is hospitalized following a nervous breakdown.

Now, let us describe the same scene in the year 2025. The case will be identical, but this time there will be Social and Medical Information Banks and a specialist – a Social Information scientist – who will help those in distress find their way through the vast maze of information available, and choose what is relevant to their needs. Let us return to Mrs Jones: immediately after her divorce she turns to the local information adviser – this will be standard procedure in the 21st century. This adviser, who will be called an ***SI scientist***, a neutral person who is neither a physician nor a psychologist, explains the possible alternatives – in this case, he suggests either psychological counseling or a support group. Mrs Jones chooses the support group, and in this way makes new friends with whom she shares common concerns. In the framework of the support group, and in addition to the regular meetings and social get-togethers, the participants occasionally conduct discussions on books, stories, or poems pertaining to divorce. Some of the participants read the books beforehand on their home computers while others prefer to hear them with the help of an electronic talking book; Mrs Jones is old-fashioned and reads the books in print. From the meetings and readings she learns about the influence of divorce on the family, different ways to alleviate the situation, and how to be more understanding and open.

Mrs Jones begins to feel more sure of herself; she goes out socializing and meets with friends. It is still hard for her, but she is coping and in control. When a problem comes up with her six-year-old son Jimmy, who seems to lack motivation and does not want to go to school, she again applies to the Social Information Bank. The adviser suggests several possibilities: he refers her to the school guidance counsellor, to a social psychologist, a neurologist, and an eye doctor to check for a possible eye problem or dyslexia. Mrs Jones does not feel helpless, she has a plan of action. She chooses to meet with the school guidance counsellor and then with a physician, who identifies the problem as dyslexia. Mrs Jones is alarmed and in need of further information, so she revisits the Social Information adviser. This time she is given a list of scientific literature about dyslexia as well as a story about a child coping with the condition.

Mrs Jones learns that it is possible to deal with her son's problem, that it is not a mental problem but that he needs support, encouragement, and opportunities for open communication with his friends in areas that do not involve reading. In her search for appropriate material to help her son, Mrs Jones returns to the ***SI scientist***, who points to the existence of an abundance of "talking books" that will enable her son to learn most of his school subjects by listening. This is acceptable to

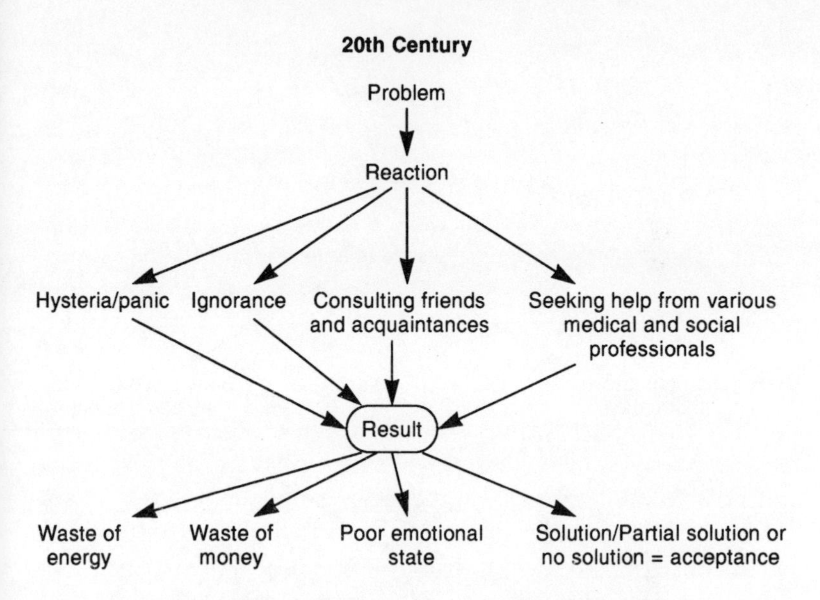

Coping with Problems – Some Basic Characteristics

Mrs Jones – it will prevent the boy from becoming cut off from society. The Jones family is in full control, and is coping calmly with the problem, rather than from a position of ignorance.

When Mrs Jones's mother suffers a stroke, she unhesitatingly turns to the Social Information Bank. She is already experienced in the procedure, and requests a book about the symptoms related to the disease. The counselor also recommends a volunteer aid organization which supplies volunteers who provide assistance for a small fee. Mrs Jones makes enquiries as to organizations which rent out wheelchairs. She now understands that her mother's negative reactions are related to the illness and that she need not take them personally. Mrs Jones is in distress, but is able to see things objectively. When the situation worsens, she turns to the Social Information Bank, receives a list of suitable institutions, enquires about the social rights to which she is entitled, and successfully has her mother admitted to a suitable nursing home. The daughter, Anne, who is fifteen at the time, is frustrated. Her mother notices this and tries to help by enrolling her talented daughter in art courses in

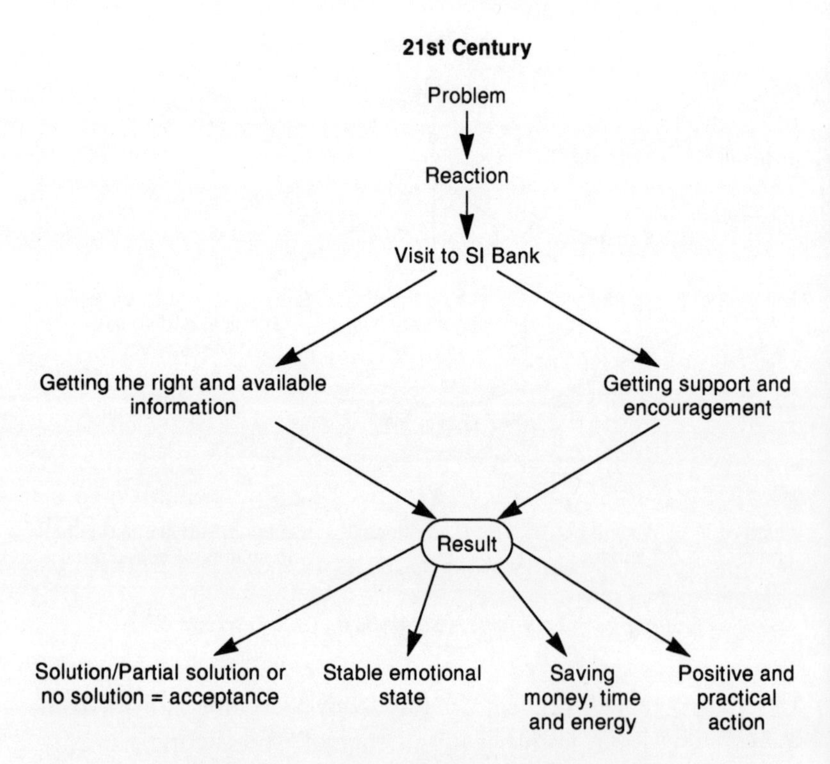

Coping with Problems – Some Basic Characteristics

order to channel her activities in a positive direction. She is only partially successful in this, and her daughter begins using drugs. Mrs Jones again turns to the Social Information Bank in search of a suitable psychologist and drug rehabilitation program. She does not become hysterical – she is in control of the situation, and knows where to turn for help. The daughter is properly treated, joins a drug rehabilitation program, and later becomes a counselor in a rehabilitated addicts' support group. By the end of the year, despite some serious problems, Mrs Jones is still functioning fully in the dual capacity of mother and daughter, she manages her life with the help of clear and explicit knowledge about her condition and the tools available for her use to improve her situation.

What we have seen is the same case – 30 years later. The problems have not changed, nor have the methods of treatment.

But Mrs Jones has much more information at her disposal. Had she lived in the year 2025 and not 1995, she would have been a lot better off.

This is a single example of the importance of the use of the right data, books, and technology. Are we moving toward a society in which the individual will have the basic tools necessary to cope? Or are we becoming a society in which information retrieval will be cold, sophisticated, and impressively efficient, yet will be unable to help the ordinary person who merely needs support, encouragement, and appropriate information. The choice is up to us. If we get it right the 21st century can herald a new interdisciplinary approach, combining basic human needs and sophisticated technology. We are already well aware of the importance of the information to be found in literature and electronic communications, as we shall see in the next chapter. However, members society in the 21st century will have to realize that sophisticated technology by itself is not enough; sensitive means of communication that will facilitate access and give assistance to all in need of aid, support, and relief will have to be invented. With a deeper awareness of the social aspects of information and literature, people like Mrs Jones should be able to find their way even before the year 2025.[1]

4

The Heritage of the 20th Century

The concept of using information and literature for the benefit of mankind is not new. The ancient Greeks called their libraries "The Healing Place for the Soul"; Muslims read the Koran in hospitals to encourage the patients; Christians draw strength and comfort from the Old and New Testaments; and Jews are never separated from their prayer books and the Book of Psalms. The 20th century has witnessed the development of official techniques and aid projects using the written word. This has been largely due to the growth of public libraries, and to the awareness of the need for support emphasized by psychologists, social workers, and educational counselors.

Today, approaching the end of the 20th century, we have basic theories and a selection of practical applications for the beneficial use of literature and information. These applications are most important – they are the fruits of the awareness of society's needs, as well as a recognition of the importance of modern technology. The only problem is that most of these activities are conducted in frameworks isolated from one another, and are not sufficiently known to the general public. Below is a brief review of the main activities in this area over the past century.

Bibliotherapy and Psychoneuroimmunology

The main field in which books and information are used for beneficial purposes is bibliotherapy. This discipline originated at the end of the 18th century, when a number of European humanitarians proposed the use of books for recreational purposes. By the beginning of the 19th century these reforms had spread to America, and Dr Benjamin Rush became the first American to recommend reading for the sick and mentally ill. He advocated the use of fiction as well as religious material. Another American physician, John Minson Galt II, wrote a seminal article on bibliotherapy in 1846. In 1904 Kathleen E. Jones, Library Administrator at McLean Hospital in Waverly, Massachusetts, became the first trained and qualified librarian to use books in a hospital framework. As a result of her efforts, bibliotherapy received its initial recognition as an aspect of librarianship. The development of bibliotherapy received great impetus during World War I in the libraries of the army hospitals and, since then, the Veterans Administration (VA) has played a significant role in its progress. It was not until the 1930s that the concept of bibliotherapy began to flourish. At that time the brothers Dr Karl and Dr William Menniger were becoming known, both through their publications and through their successful psychiatric practice in the Menniger Clinic, where much of the work with patients was based on the use of carefully selected extracts from books. The patients were assigned specific titles to read, which they would then discuss with their psychiatrist in relation to their own problems. By 1939 the Hospital Division of the American Library Association (ALA) had established a Bibliotherapy Committee for the purpose of studying bibliotherapy. Bibliotherapy had finally achieved "official" status in librarianship.[1]

The 1940s, '50s, and '60s produced research and publications on the use of bibliotherapy as related to specific emotional needs. The most important work of this period was Caroline Shrodes's doctoral dissertation, "Bibliotherapy, a Theoretical and Clinical Experimental Study" (1949), which provided a psychological framework for the dynamics of bibliotherapy.[2] By 1961 two of the better known authoritative dictionaries – *Webster's Third New International Dictionary* and *The Random House Dictionary* – included definitions of the term "bibliotherapy." The former was: "The use of selected reading material as therapeutic adjuncts in medicine and psychiatry,

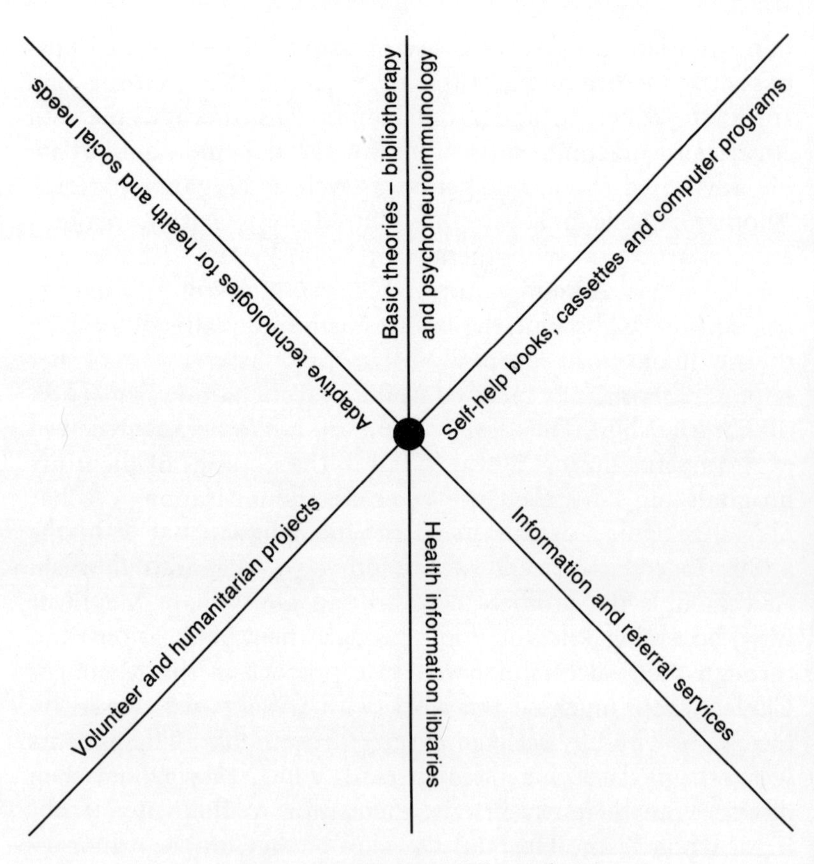

Six Angles – the Heritage of the 20th Century

also guidance in the solution of personal problems through directed reading"; Random House's definition was: "The use of reading as an ameliorative adjunct to therapy." The most recent definition of bibliotherapy can be found in Barker's recently-published *Social Work Dictionary* (1987): "The use of literature and poetry in treatment of people with emotional problems or mental illness. Bibliotherapy is often used in social group work and group therapy, and is reported to be effective with people of all ages, with people in institutions as well as outpatients, and with healthy people who wish to share literature as a means of personal growth and development."[3]

Many dedicated scholars have contributed to the development of bibliotherapy in the fields of psychology and librarianship, such as R. Rubin (1978), E. F. Brown (1975), and Pardeck and Pardeck (1984, 1993). However, the person credited with creating the practical concept of modern bibliotherapy is Arleen McCarty Hynes, who established the first hospital-based training program in bibliotherapy in 1974 at St Elizabeth's Psychiatric Hospital in Washington. Her major contribution to the field is her well-known book: *Biblio/Poetry Therapy – The Interactive Process* (1986), which was designed to teach how the whole spectrum of literature – from poetry to science fiction – could be used to promote greater self-knowledge, to renew the spirit and, in general, to aid the healing process. Arleen McCarty Hynes also developed bibliotherapy workshops, study programs, and volunteer organizations.

The increasing awareness of the hidden potential of books has initiated academic research in the fields of psychology, education, social work, and librarianship. To date, several hundred research studies in this field have been published in the western world and in eastern Europe. Most of them indicate that the bibliotherapeutic process can effect positive change in the person being treated. Bibliotherapy has been found to be helpful in changing attitudes, in bringing about behavioral change, in reducing fear, and in revealing a patient's hidden potential. Nevertheless one of the essential criticisms of bibliotherapy is that it is not an exact science, and some researchers are skeptical about its possible results, as Pardeck and Pardeck (1993) indicated:

> What should be noted however is that virtually all of the helping therapies are far from exact. Bibliotherapy is no exception. Bibliotherapy may be more complex than other therapies because one must be skilled both in selecting literature that parallels the problem facing a client and in knowing how to use such literature as a therapeutic medium. If one can combine these steps successfully, bibliotherapy can provide a very valuable treatment approach.[4]

I have no intention here of discussing the degree to which bibliotherapy does or does not help; what is clear is that even if the help is minimal – and involves only moral support, a kind word, or practical advice to an individual in distress – it does justify the development of this new field. Even if the reading merely serves as a distraction or a new kind of communication between parent and child, its existence is still of maximal importance.

Bibliotherapy can now be studied in the framework of the social sciences, and also in a small number of Librarianship and Information Studies departments, for example, at the University of South Florida in the USA, and at Bar-Ilan University in Israel, where the author of this book has developed a special program called "Information and Society – Facilitative Librarianship," of which bibliotherapy is one of the main branches. In the United States, the profession is also taught in private workshops, as well as organized workshops sponsored by the American Library Association (ALA), the National Association of Poetry Therapists (NAPT), and several other organizations, most of them voluntary.[5]

The communication channels described so far involve three factors: (a) the reader or listener, (b) the book, (c) the therapist or story-teller. However, there is another type of bond, the personal bond between man and book. A person chooses what it is he wants to read or watch. The very fact of that choice proves that man has both the need and the will to read that particular book or to watch a specific movie as opposed to another.

In Y. Gold's brilliant study entitled *Read for your Life* (1990), he explains how reading is essential to our basic existence. Through reading, we are able to escape to other worlds or to forget our troubles; we cope with covert impulses such as violence and cruelty, we develop our imagination, and experience happiness and joy. In his study, Gold, for the first time, refers to "the aware reader," and suggests that the reader develop a personal bibliotherapeutic method by identifying the elements that interest or repel him or her in books and then testing them in the framework of his or her own life. According to Gold, the need to read is a basic human need, and it is irrelevant whether the book is conveyed by speech or sound.[6]

The thirst to know and to understand is an integral part of

the human personality. It is no coincidence that the world's three leading religions – Judaism, Christianity, and Islam – arose around books: the Old and New Testaments of the Bible, and the Koran. These books have accompanied human history over the centuries. They were a focal point of comfort and a wellspring where mankind could seek answers. Even if answers were not always to be found, they still allowed people to feel that they were not alone, that they had someone to turn to, and something to think about. Literature and information are basic tools for human existence, not only for educated people but also for those unable to read and write, who can obtain accurate information from a middleman – a "story-teller" – or from any person disclosing information, or even a technological device. One of the most common phenomena illustrating how much people in the modern world still need the book and story is the growing industry of story-telling cassettes, especially in the United States. The fact that in the hectic, fast-flowing, and stressful times in which we live, people still take the time and have the desire to listen to a story told in the style of the ancient story-tellers, proves that "story-telling cassettes" fulfill one of our basic needs.[7]

Further testimony to the importance of the story for the human soul is its use in therapeutic methods such as "neurolinguistic programming" (NLP), whose purpose is to help people change using human behavior models (linguistic, strategic, and body language). In this method, stories are used to modify the subconsciousness using different hypnotic techniques. The idea here is that it is possible to create a connection with the subconscious, not with logical argument but through indirect symbols such as stories. As the subconscious communicates with us through indirect symbols such as those which we experience in dreams, so we can communicate with our subconscious using the same tool.[8] This theory is particularly evident in the hypnotic techniques of Milton H. Erickson, as described in his well-known book *My Voice Will Go with You – The Teaching Tales of Milton H. Erickson* (1982). If the hidden roles played by bibliotherapy, story-telling, and Erickson's hypnosis are revealed, a link is created between mankind and his soul – a link that has hitherto been mislaid somewhere along the way in humanity's struggle to understand and to find logic in life.

Having the appropriate information and the right book can help us move from an emotional state of confusion and helplessness to a position where we have more understanding and insight, to a new approach, and, sometimes, to a point when we are able to take control of the situation and plan a strategy of action. In effect, all these elements point to emotional transformation from a state of helplessness to one of understanding and action.

The 20th century has been the first to scientifically investigate the influence of our emotional state on our immune system. This new science is called psychoneuroimmunology, and was developed at the University of California in Los Angeles (UCLA). Today there is scientific evidence, based on comparative tests, that a person's emotional state has a significant influence on his or her immune system and the healing ability of the body. The new term "psychoneuroimmunology" describes the complex reciprocal interactions between the nervous system, the endocrine system, and the immune system. A picture is emerging from the many new studies being conducted which illustrates the manner in which ideas, experiences, and attitudes can create biological change. There are people who are "cured" by being given placebos, while others become depressed or suffer from a collapsed immune system due to anxiety. Yelling "Fire" in a crowded hall can spark a wide range of physiological effects, including sudden increases in blood pressure and of adrenalin. It is a known fact, for instance, that the level of cholesterol in accountants rises as the deadline for tax reports nears. Similar physiological changes appear in many students preparing for their final exams. Prominent researchers of the connection between the spirit and the immune system, immunologist Dr Ronald Glaser and psychologist Janice Kicolt Glaser of the Ohio State University Medical College, have discovered that as final exams in medicine draw near, the students display a marked decrease in the number of immunizing, disease-fighting cells, as well as damaging changes to immune system organs. It is now recognized that laughter, humor, and a supportive environment play an important role in emotional balance.[9]

At first glance, psychoneuroimmunology seems to be unrelated to either information or literature, which are – after all – the subject-matter of this book. However, in effect, psychoneuroimmunology is the major scientific premise given to us by the 20th century for justifying the importance of developing an awareness of the use of information and literature for the benefit of mankind. We have always known that a kind word, comfort, and "joie de vivre" can help people get through difficult situations. The 20th century, however, has thoroughly investigated this phenomenon and has given scientific approval to this assumption. It is up to us to develop the various ways in which psychoneuroimmunology can be applied to modern society, aided by the fields of Information, literature, and advanced technology.

Self-help Books, Cassettes, Computer Programs

The unique conditions and ambience of the 20th century have caused many individuals to suffer an identity crisis. The new means of communication have exposed the modern world to innovative ideas, but also to unknown phenomena. The old world of yesterday has begun to crumble, and people have begun to seek their true identity, such as the "flower children," the mystic cults, those seeking happiness through drugs, or the "back to nature" trends which put emphasis on healthy nutrition and positive thinking. This combination of technological and spiritual elements has created a unique atmosphere where personal solutions and new alternatives are sought. Book publishers have integrated into this special atmosphere by publishing a large number of "self-help books," ranging from self-help guides, to popular research books about the psychology of the human soul. These books were designed to give the information and tools necessary for self-improvement and better health. Among such publications are books on popular psychology, diet and exercise guides, pregnancy guides, guides for diabetics and cancer patients, and popular literature for improving one's lifestyle and understanding the importance of preventive medicine. According to Rees (1991), in his study about managing consumer health information services, more than one thousand books are published annually in the United States for the lay reader interested in health-care topics.[10] The publishers not only deal with health issues, but also produce many books and cassettes on mysticism, astrology, Eastern philosophy, meditation, yoga, etc. Over the last few years we have also witnessed the flourishing of technical life-improvement aids, such as relaxation and biofeedback cassettes, biofeedback computer programs, and the initial aid data bases, such as the "Combined Health Information" (CHID), which contains references to consumer health information and promotion material, including formally published peripheral literature and audiovisual material. Also included are health promotion projects currently in process in the United States.

The awareness of the importance of aid information is also slowly penetrating into the field of portable data bases (information on floppy disks or CD-Rom), for example the British "Helpbox," which includes the most comprehensive coverage of British consumer health information. Self-help information is a widespread phenomenon, as the "health and lifestyle columns" in the popular press show. The development of the concept of preventive medicine is also related to this general trend. All these phenomena indicate that we, on the brink of the 21st century, are interested in seeking personal solutions and information that will help us improve our lifestyle.[11]

Information and Referral Services

Institutions for the provision of information, both for aid and for welfare, have been set up within different frameworks, such as government and municipal offices, and public libraries. These institutions were established to help the public and guide it through the bureaucratic maze of social and health issues. Since the publication of *Neighborhood Information Centers: A Study and Some Proposals* (1966), by Alfred J. Kahn *et al.*, the interest in establishing Information and Referral Services (I&RS) has grown rapidly. Kahn and his colleagues analyzed the structure and activities of the "British Citizens Advice Bureau" (CAB); they noted the lack of anything similar in the United States, and proposed alternative means. As part of the growing interest in the social aspect of information, many institutions have become concerned with creating a switching center that can link an individual – whatever his or her need – with an appropriate resource. T. Childers, in his study on Information and Referral Services in public libraries (1983), explains that existing agencies, such as the health and welfare councils in many cities, have sometimes taken on this function. In addition, a number of new organizations have developed, such as Search in Los Angeles, the Model Cities Community Information Center in Philadelphia, and Operation Communication in Wilmington.[12]

The public libraries joined this trend in the 1960s, and many public libraries in the United States now house an I&RS section. In reality, the great majority of them are not as widely known to the general public as they should be. One of the reasons for this, as Childers indicates, is the fact that most I&RS are intended for deprived persons, and very few have been developed to address the needs of the "average" person. That is why the I&RS sometimes bears the stigma of servicing mainly the poor and deprived.[13] Another example which indicates modern society's desire to be informed about social problems and health information is the establishment of the Public College of Health, set up in 1983. This is a British non-profit organization under the jurisdiction of the Consumers' Association. Its function is to supply the public with health-related information services.[14]

There is no doubt that the activities of the I&RS over the past 30 years merit social recognition and should be more thoroughly researched. It is unfortunate that activity of such significance should sometimes be hidden from view, and does not receive the social recognition it deserves. If scientific cooperation between these various organizations could be cultivated, a great deal would be learned from their experiences, failures, and successes. We would have been able to research such subjects as the informational needs of the public, the best types of service to fill those needs, funding, links with health care and social institutional staff, location of services, levels and type of staff, information resources, equipment, and publicity. The vast experience acquired in I&RS could form a solid base for the development of information aid centers in the 21st century.

Health Information Libraries

There is also growing awareness of the need for information in the official institutions which treat patients. In a survey among US hospitals, conducted by the American Hospital Association (AHA) in 1987, it was found that 21.4 percent of the hospitals which responded to the questionnaires had Health Information Libraries, also known as Library Resource Centers. The institutions which were pioneers in this field were Lenox Hill Hospital in New York and the Kaiser Oakland Health Maintenance Organization in California. The 1987 AHA survey shows that providing information is the most important aspect of all the above mentioned centers. They all have three major goals in common:

- To inform – to supply current information on health, disease, and well-being in spoken/written form and through the media, so that the consumer can understand and use it.
- To teach – to provide opportunities for the consumer to learn the skills of self-care, self-management, and coping with health problems.
- To promote the hospital – to offer information that will help the consumer make better and more positive links with the hospital, its medical staff, and other health-care providers.

The consumers in these hospitals can gain access to information in two ways: (a) by the consumers walking into the library and either browsing or asking for help; (b) by telephoning the center and asking a specific question, and receiving the answer either on the spot or by mail. The staff members, when needed, put the consumer in touch with a health-care provider in the hospital or outside it, such as a pharmacist or nutritionist. In addition, when necessary, the consumer is referred to a community, state, or nationally organized support group. These referrals are often managed by computerized programs that permit the resource center's staff to give the consumer a choice of several appropriate physicians or information about the possible alternatives.

The establishment of information centers in hospitals has come about as a response to public demand. In one such center, the Planetree Health Resource Center in San Francisco, the staff often prepare as many as one hundred information packages a month in response to requests by the public.

Robin Orr, the National Director of Hospital Projects for Planetree, says:

> Health professionals don't need to protect consumers from information. In fact, the best way to empower and enable consumers of health-care services is to freely give them access to information that will help them make good choices.[15]

Volunteer and Humanitarian Projects

Help through the reading of books has become a part of the activities of volunteer groups which have been set up specifically to offer assistance and support. There are two important, humanitarian projects that can serve as a model for other projects, being of benefit to those in need as well as to the volunteers themselves.

The first project is the "Book Buddies program" which is run in the hospitals of San Francisco. This program actually began in October 1985 with the backing of a Library Services and Construction Act (LSCA) grant of $120,000, which covered the cost of the book collection and in-service training workshops.

The underlying idea behind this program is that children and their families coping with hospital stays can be therapeutically helped by being told stories. To make this service available to the young patient, the San Francisco Public Library trains approximately 120 new Book Buddies a year. These volunteers read to over 4,000 children in seven hospitals, and also to the children visiting pediatric outpatient clinics. This is an ideal opportunity for the children to experience the warmth and comfort of a "read aloud" session, and also provides an excellent opportunity to introduce the library services to children and their families.

Potential Book Buddies are interviewed by the hospital staff and undergo health screening before being accepted. The volunteers chosen are then trained in a special one-day program on subjects such as the hospital environment, the importance of story-telling, the difficulties of reading books in a medically active environment, children's literature, and techniques for sharing books with children. Maintaining the link between the volunteers and the library is very important. This is accomplished through in-service training events, distribution of a newsletter, the bestowing of recognition awards, and the holding of special events for volunteers. To help identify the program, the library volunteers wear a Book Buddies' button and carry a Book Buddies' bag. Each Book Buddies' location maintains a collection of approximately 600 books donated by the library. In order to reflect the needs of San Francisco's diverse communities, approximately 15 percent of the books are in Chinese, Spanish, and Vietnamese. Collections include story-telling support material, such as hand and finger puppets, and a flannel board with pre-cut story figures. Much can be learned from this unique program, which brings so much love to the children – and a feeling of fulfillment for the volunteers.[16]

The second service which deserves mention is a fascinating German project called "*Das Frohliche Krankenzimmer*," or, in English: "The Happy Children's Ward." The pilot project was formed in 1981 to test bibliotherapeutic principles in a children's clinic. The project corresponded to the general goals of the hospital reform movement then gaining momentum: making the hospital environment more humane for young patients. The medium, or "instruments," chosen by the project for accomplishing this goal were carefully selected books. Since these goals were strongly supported by the German Medical Women's Association, this organization became the official sponsor of the program and the late Dr Edith Mundt MD took charge of coordinating this innovative project.

For 13 years prior to this, the German Association for Children's Literature had been sending "Happy Children's Ward"-book parcels to pediatric hospitals. It was intuitively reasoned that "happy children get well faster." This assumption has since been scientifically supported by research in the field of psychoneuroimmunology. However, there was no direct contact with the children in hospital who were presumed to be reading the books, nor with the hospital staff who were supposedly reading the books to the children. More direct feedback was needed.

In 1981 the Dr von Hauner's Children's Clinic of the University of Munich provided a working environment for the project. Collection and organization of books donated by the German Association for Children's Literature and German publishers formed the basis of the outreach to the children's wards. Medical personnel were initially wary of having "outsiders" bring books to the hospitalized children, and much time and effort was expended in ensuring hygienic control of the books. As the medical staff became increasingly aware of the positive psychophysical effects of the patient interaction with the stories contained in the books, the antiseptic issue became less acute. For example, children being read a story during preoperative preparations were far less distressed; children who read books or who had books read to them were less demanding of the nurses' attention. Intensive interaction between children and books could also provide important diagnostic and rehabilitative information. It was found that formerly noncommunicative patients initiated conversations based on pertinent story incidents – sometimes in conjunction with symptom-disclosure statements. Observing parent–book–child interactions also added significant details to behavioral reports. Such information was particularly well received by those medical personnel accepting a biopsychosocial model of the child. Following the overwhelmingly positive reception in Munich, sub-groups were formed. Members of the German Medical Women's Association, already active in clinics all over Germany, were contacted to form and oversee these sub-groups.

In order to be able to contribute scientifically-based evidence on the effects of books in a hospital setting, Dr Carol Adeney carried out empirical research between 1983 and 1987. Picture books with either a proven or a postulated beneficial therapeutic effect in the hospital setting were regularly read to, and discussed with, chronically ill youngsters for the duration of their hospital stay. Under certain conditions, the following results were observed: the adult–child contact was enhanced through the mere presence of a book; the attention span of adult and child was increased when book-centered; the child's interest in the information conveyed by the book or its metaphoric theme was enhanced through adult input related to the book; the child exhibited more vitality during and after being read to from an appropriate book; the adult–child interaction was more relaxed when book-centered; the adult–child interaction was more emotionally expressive when book-centered; the child desired the interaction to continue; the child complained less of being in pain while reading a book or being read to; the child's complaints of homesickness were reduced; the child was less fearful; the child's complaints of being bored decreased; and the child's positive memories of his/her hospital experience were enhanced.

In the absence of a systematic data base, books were chosen from the "Happy Children's Ward's" pool of experience. Such a data base would certainly increase the effectiveness of attempts to match a child's needs, inner world, and interests with a particular book's presentation. The German Medical Women's Association has attempted to bridge the gap between an individual sharing of "favorite" therapeutic books and a systematic inventory of therapeutic literature. Since 1975 it has awarded "The Silver Feather" to fiction or non-fiction books dealing with well-being and illness, and has thus contributed to the increased production of such books. In addition, "The Happy

Children's Ward" pilot project has published a catalog (now in its 4th revised edition) of recommended books – both fiction and non-fiction – for children in hospital and for personnel working with children in hospital.[17]

Adaptive Technologies for Health/Social Needs

In addition to basic theories and practical social projects, information-storing technology has been used during the past century as a method of improving the lifestyle of the blind, the deaf, and those with motor and speech impairments. Although these problems cannot be prevented, life can be made better, and people can be helped to function in the society of which they are part. An important review of information technology in the field of aid is to be found in Joseph J. Lazzaro's comprehensive book (1993), which is recommended to anyone planning to work with social information.

Many of the difficulties faced by the blind or the visually impaired can nowadays be reduced through adaptive technologies, mainly with the help of a personal computer. Talking computer systems can be programmed to verbalize keystrokes and information displayed on the screen. With the assistance of a talking computer, blind people can read and write, study, and manage business and personal affairs; they can have access to information data bases and manage financial resources. In addition, there are magnification systems that can now enlarge the print in books and other printed documents on the computer screen, and publishers of documents in Braille can work hand-in-hand with most computer systems.

For the deaf or people with hearing problems, the text telephone allows them to "talk" on the telephone using keyboards and printers to send messages back and forth. Captioning systems allow equal access to video programming, providing text messages for the audio portion of programming.

Another group that can benefit from the new information technologies are those with motor or speech impairments. Computers can now be adapted to respond to spoken commands.

Adapted keyboards can be customized for persons with minimal typing ability, and special switches can respond to any body movement. For those who have no voice, there are portable communication devices that can speak, and for those who have motor impairments, there are environmental systems that can turn electronic equipment on and off, and control heating and lighting systems.[18]

The social activities and innovations mentioned above are all important, but equally important is the public's awareness of the basic fact that information, literature, and technology can be of assistance. The necessary knowledge and tools to obtain help from all the information resources developed by mankind is on the verge of being universally available. As we approach the 21st century we have two options: the first is to continue to develop independent projects, without any particular unifying direction and without the possibility of direct and immediate access between one and another. This allows the existing state to continue as it is; it grants freedom of creativity in the belief that whatever is built will be used in a constructive manner. By this process, there would be continued development of specialized computer programs, local and national aid programs, and it would be possible to read books in a variety of ways – on computer screens, with a giant projector, or with the help of a talking book. In addition, data bases to be constructed would include vast amounts of information that would be potentially of benefit. This vast concentration of information could be schematically divided into major categories, such as industrial, commercial, educational, medical information, etc. Despite the importance of all these activities, this information – with its huge potential to help society – would be scattered and dispersed throughout these diverse projects and networks just as it is today, far from those people who need it most. Why should the citizens of the 21st century be denied the use of this information and the existing tools for aid in a simple and straightforward manner, for their own benefit and that of their families?

This brings us to our second option, which is to develop new ways of thinking, to extricate the possible aid factors from the huge network of "information, literature, and technology," and to develop a mutually enriching relationship between projects, researchers, and human needs.

Such a positive and constructive approach calls for an interdisciplinary and original outlook. This is not fantasy or a project beyond human knowledge, but rather a simple mission to increase the awareness of the *existing* positive and constructive tools, and to develop and adapt them for the common good. A consensus exists in today's world as to the use of arms – destructive arms such as nuclear weapons are restricted and controlled. Why should there not be a consensus concerning the importance of developing all means of aiding and benefitting the human race? Such a consensus could be shared by, and be acceptable to, all religions and political outlooks. The simple fact is that human history has endowed us with information, literature, and technology that can improve our lives; once this is recognized it follows that we should think how the various components of this knowledge can be combined for the welfare of humanity. A new scientific discipline – "Social Information Science" – will integrate all the components and lead to the development of scientific research and practical applications. The world has a treasure in its possession, but insight and initiative are necessary for it to be utilized and developed in a positive and creative way.

5

A New Scientific Discipline

In general, it is the needs of society which dictate the creation of new professions and disciplines. During the late 19th and the 20th centuries we witnessed the rise of many new academic disciplines, among them sociology, anthropology, psychology, demography, criminology, economy, business management, political science, genetics, and others. Each of these professions was created in order to address special needs of the human race and to improve the life of modern society.

The 20th century moved away from the conservative European-style universities, which catered only to the elite and concentrated on the traditional established academic subjects, such as philosophy, literature, history, languages, medicine, and the natural sciences. With the 20th century came a major change in academic consumption: the human race and its social and emotional needs became the subject for research, an object to be studied and improved. Today, just a few years before the millennium, the new task is to develop professions that will be attentive and sensitive to modern needs. The task now is to reveal all the "hidden" sources that can help us, and this can only be done through the establishment of a new scientific discipline – "Social Information Science." The purpose of this new academic branch will be to "locate" all the beneficial elements found within the huge pool of existing information and literature, to investigate their influence on society, and to develop new social applications.

In the 21st century, people coping with a specific problem will turn to the Social Information Bank, where they will be provided with clear and reliable information. In the bank they will find details about organizations which can assist them, support groups, types of treatment, and literature, poetry and films that can provide them with some support and understanding.

In this way, in the coming century, anyone with a problem – however large or small – will be able to get initial guidance to begin coping with his or her problem, and to use the support tools available for the specific situation. As the profession of "Social Information Scientist" becomes more clearly defined, the public will gradually become more aware of its potential, and will use more and more information. It is easy to categorize such help in terms of small project developments. But the development of hundreds and thousands of such small projects, without their being defined in the framework of a specific profession, will miss out on the potential; the number of electronic and communications programs will increase, but the result will be an unstructured and unfocused mass of information. Only when central "Social Information Banks," operating on an objective scientific basis, are established, will the new discipline be able to make a real contribution to Society.

People will gradually become aware that in these new banks there is someone who can understand their problems, needs, and limitations, someone familiar with literature, books, information and electronic communications, someone who is neutral and not emotionally involved – whose only job is to give the most reliable information available in as short a time as possible. The Social Information Banks will, thus, become a routine part of life in the 21st century. The people of the 21st century will know that the center will be able to access the best available information as to who is most suited to deal with the problem: a psychologist, physician, or social worker. The location, address, and telephone numbers of institutions or appropriate therapists will be supplied, and the enquiring individuals will be told if they are entitled to assistance or financial aid. They will also receive printed information dealing with their problem and ways to cope with it; they will leave the Bank with information on relevant literature, films, and support groups. These individuals will always be free to return to the Social Information

Bank to seek additional information if or when a new problem or complication crops up. The people of the 21st century will be free to choose the most suitable alternatives and will be sure that, through the Social Information Bank, they have access to most of the available tools for help.

One of the psychological results will be a lessening of the feeling of total helplessness during times of stress and crisis. People will become aware that they have some freedom of choice in the selection of the most suitable alternatives. In this way humanity will become more self-aware and thus more mature.

The scenario outlined above is not a call to change the current social and therapeutic establishment: those satisfied with the conventional approach and who are not interested in trying something different will continue as before; others may find that the new approach suits them and their lifestyle, and they will be able to take full advantage of it. The old social establishment will also be able to use the services of the new Social Information Bank. They will have the opportunity to be connected by network to this Bank and, in this way, to reduce red tape and concentrate on giving the best treatment and service to the person in need.

The obvious question that comes to mind is how to begin. Most academic disciplines develop spontaneously according to the creativity of the scholars and the needs of society. The new discipline of Social Information should not be any different, but since we are talking about an interdisciplinary field of science that connects scholars from different academic disciplines and various practical professions, it is in order to recommend some initial first steps. As we live in an advanced technological era, perhaps the first thing to do is to start building an electronic discussion group for all scholars interested in "Social Information Science." In addition to spontaneous group discussions, work should begin on the first "Social Information data base," which will be built up gradually by a steady stream of information coming from scholars, organizations, and universities.

Why a data base? In order to build such a new interdisciplinary profession, basic information on the subject must be located, categorized, and defined. Only then can SI theories and new practical applications be developed. Establishing the new discipline would involve the following five important components for helping people:

I Direct and hidden information
II Literature and poetry
III Practical ongoing projects
IV Theoretical studies
V Academic curriculum.

I. Direct Information and Hidden Information

Included in this category is a large amount of information contained in books, articles, cassettes, and films. For example: on "do-it-yourself" diet; healthy pregnancy, and child-raising guides, etc.; directories of addresses for health and welfare services; guides to aid organizations; cassettes for relaxation and guided imagination; films about preventive medicine, such as how to avoid Aids, how to quit smoking, and so on; government-published brochures and pamphlets which are distributed in health clinics and hospitals; and television programs dealing with health issues. In addition to direct information, other information is now only available after a thorough and sometimes complicated search, for example: accurate medical information contained in scientific as well as popular journals; civil rights issues concealed in government publications, names of unlisted organizations and support groups, etc. The data base need not include all the literature on the above subjects but there should be enough basic material that will enable scholars and Social Information Scientists to start to build a basic collection of tools for their social data banks.[1]

II. Literature and Poetry

Within the discipline of bibliotherapy, bibliographical lists have been compiled containing recommended literature dealing with health and social problems. Most of these lists were compiled in the United States – a partial list can be found in Arleen

Hynes's study on bibliotherapy. The lists are divided into sections representing different health and social problems, and can be used when a direct approach to a problem is needed. The use of such literary works is called direct bibliotherapy; for example, recommending to a divorced father a certain book about the way another divorced father has coped. While all literature and poetry can serve as a tool for aid and support if they fit the person's inner world, "indirect" bibliotherapy tools cannot be categorized in perfect ready-made lists. What is possible, however, is to integrate the "direct bibliotherapy lists" in order to help the Social Information scientists, librarians, and aid professionals using literature in their work.[2]

III. Practical Ongoing Projects

I include here all ongoing projects which use the entire media means available for assistance and support: official and volunteer projects in hospitals, such as San Francisco's "Book Buddies," support groups, aid organizations, the information and referral services in public libraries, information centers in hospitals, and projects developing advanced technology for helping people. Once a pool of such projects is developed there can be interaction and discussion between the project managers, thus creating new initiatives and contributing to the development of the new field of Social Information.[3]

IV. Theoretical Studies

This category includes all the research literature investigating the use of literature and the media for aid purposes. This information is not concentrated under one roof but is found in different disciplines, mostly with no connection between them. We find such studies in the following scientific branches: bibliotherapy, librarianship, preventive medicine, psychology, rehabilitation and welfare, and social science. The correlation of such studies will shed light and inspire new ideas about the way that literature and information can help.[4]

V. Academic Curriculum

As of today, there is no defined discipline which teaches Social Information in a direct and authoritative manner. However, there are several schools of librarianship, such as the University of California, which do teach bibliotherapy. There are also bibliotherapy workshops in the United States. In Bar-Ilan University in Israel, where I currently head the Information Studies and Librarianship Department, I have developed a unique program named "Information and Society – Facilitative Librarianship." In addition, courses on preventive medicine and patient education, which are sometimes given in social science departments and medical schools, are ideal for instituting a Social Information ethic and working pattern. The interaction between the scholars that head these courses can lead to the building of a solid base for developing Social Information specialization in universities.[5]

The five categories mentioned above are the first which come to mind when studying human knowledge as a source of help and support. Just as archeologists sometimes discover new and unexpected findings, so it is possible that those dealing with this new profession will find a much more valuable treasure after initial trials.

The task of locating existing material is not an easy one, and it necessitates sophisticated searching techniques through all the available sources: books, directories, reference literature, data bases, and electronic group discussion. An interesting interaction between all the factors in the system can be reached using the new electronic means available today. Links may develop between researchers working on different projects who, as yet, are unaware of each other's existence. The first to benefit are people – the information consumers – who will be able to receive the necessary information and help more quickly. The therapeutic sector will receive new working tools; hospitals, rehabilitation, and aid centers will be able to consult each other and exchange information and assistance. Even if we can not yet envision the day when this major project will be completed, the potential benefits can be easily assessed in the light of present-day social policies and currently available technology.

Cultural Policy

Who, then, is going to undertake this mission of starting a discussion group and building the new data base? Who is qualified to take on such a project? In some countries it could be the Departments of Welfare or Health, or international organizations such as UNESCO, or the Red Cross. If it is not done on a national or international scale, then, at the very least, it has to be done on a small scale by people familiar with the information field and social needs. Organizations such as the American Library Association (ALA) and the International Federation of Library Associations and Institutions (IFLA) would be ideal candidates, as their personnel would recognize the significance and worthiness of this project. Similarly, schools of information and librarianship would be ideal, and it would be a natural development to set up courses of study for the new field of Social Information. In recent years, librarianship departments have had to deal with the problem of the entry of business and computer-trained personnel into the field of information retrieval; sometimes this has resulted in the closing of departments. This trend could be reversed once librarianship departments were appraised of the importance of Supportive and Social Information, and the possible integration of technological tools into the social aspects of human needs. Under these circumstances, additional schools of librarianship and information would open.[6]

Some wishful thinking: Since the American government is one of the leading nations in advanced technology, as is shown in the "superhighway" project, it would be ideally placed to initiate the establishment of the "Foundation for Social Information Science," in collaboration with the high-tech companies and representatives of all nations seeking peace and well-being. This foundation would enable qualified people from the fields of Information Science and the Social Sciences to set up an international electronic discussion group and to build the first data base, thus supporting academic research in the new field and helping the development of practical projects.

The current American Administration is not only attentive theoretically to peace and welfare issues, but has also made real progress in the areas of health and international peace, as in the case of the Middle East. The next step toward peace and welfare might be the building of a "social international superhighway" for the benefit of all people around the world. This would be not only an important step forward for the American government and people, but a new stage in the development of the social organization of the human race.

Literature, information and high-tech are means of communication: these means can be directed toward establishing a "practical peace" between nations – not just a diplomatic peace, but a real peace in terms of helping and supporting people by the exchange of ideas and knowledge between various nations and races. Will the American "superhighway" be the initiator of this new "practical peace" and serve as the bridge between nations? Only time will tell.

6

The Future **SI Scientist**

The 20th century saw the rise not only of new academic disciplines, but also of new professions, like the psychologist, the social scientist, and the school counsellor, who use social and emotional skills to provide help and guidance to people in distress. The next century will see the creation of another new professional, the Social Information scientist, who will use a combination of advanced technologies to deal with human needs. One of the lessons learned at the end of the 20th century is that although the different fields of science have been artificially separated throughout history, they are in fact all related to each other. This conclusion has led to a tendency to develop new interdisciplinary research studies that link the different disciplines together. The new academic discipline of "Social Information Science" fits into this approach – responding to the real needs of society with the most modern and sophisticated means available.

The creation of a new profession always raises questions. What sort of person should the Social Information scientist be? Where will this individual be educated? What special training will be required? In which frameworks will the Social Information scientist be qualified to work? What will the specific duties be? What are the limitations of the profession? And, lastly, will we really need such a discipline in the age of electronic communications, when almost every family will have a computer and a modem at home?

Since the Social Information scientist will be mentioned many times, it is as well to provide a shortened name. Let us call this individual the ***SI scientist,*** not only because it is an easy name to remember, but because the positive nature of the new profession is also concealed in the word "Si" which means "yes" in a number of languages.

What Sort of Person should the *SI Scientist* be?

What are the special qualities required for a person to be a successful ***SI scientist***? The new ***SI scientists*** will have to be talented in many fields, and possess a special ability to combine these talents in a new interdisciplinary profession. To begin with, they must have a broad, general education and a basic knowledge of subjects related to social welfare and information science. They should be empathic individuals with an ability to relate to people in distress, but at the same time be able to remain emotionally uninvolved. They should be intuitive, broad-minded, and have the capacity to think analytically in order to evaluate information, understand its social potential, and relay the information to the consumer in the best way possible. They must be creative and flexible thinkers, able to quickly size up situations, and choose the information best suited for each case. In addition, the ***SI scientists*** should be familiar with information sources and methods for gathering information; they must know the advanced techniques for retrieving and organizing information, and have good organizational skills. Nowadays, in light of the advances of science and technology, we cannot expect one person to be an expert in so many fields; however, the ***SI scientist*** should be a very intelligent and sensitive person who has basic all-round knowledge in the fields mentioned above. This basic knowledge will enable him or her to operate alone, and, when necessary, to choose the appropriate expert adviser and to communicate with that individual in the most proficient way possible.

Where will the *SI Scientist* be Educated?

In order to ensure that the new discipline enters the public awareness and develops in a professional manner, an official academic curriculum is a necessity. The ***SI scientist*** must enter the job market with clear and precise knowledge, and with an academic degree in his field. The departments of "Information Studies and Librarianship" at the university level would be the ideal place for the study of "Social Information." Today, these departments train their students in all the latest technology. Most of the students accepted into their programs have BA degrees and, at the end of their studies, will have earned a certificate or a master's degree. In order to open a course of study for the exclusive training of ***SI scientists***, a special program would have to be developed that would accept only those holding BA degrees in the social sciences. This would ensure that the students had a basic knowledge and understanding of human needs. Of course, there are options for choosing other university departments for the training of ***SI scientists***, but they are not as suitable as the schools of information and librarianship. At first glance, it seems possible to train people having computer and business administration backgrounds; however, their approach is often market-oriented, which is hardly suitable for dealing with sensitive issues and people in need. The new ***SI scientist*** must be attentive to people's needs and not just be a computer expert.

Another possibility is for SI sciences to be taught in the social science departments by adding special courses in information technologies. The drawback to this proposition is the "professional motivation" of the students and teaching staff, which is often therapy-oriented. Their purpose is to provide treatment and direct assistance through their special skills. There is a possibility that while giving information they might, consciously or unconsciously, slide back into the area of therapy or their specific speciality, and unintentionally force their particular brand of training on the consumer. In addition, of course, they are more education-oriented and less information-minded; they will be somewhat unfamiliar with the vast potential of information organization systems and retrieval techniques.

The new ***SI scientist*** must be objective, an agent who is competent in giving information but by no means a therapist.

It is especially neutrality, objectiveness, and detachment that will enable people to feel that they have free choice and are not being pushed toward any particular solution. By establishing "Information Studies and Librarianship" departments, the new profession will acquire an information-oriented image rather than a therapeutic one, and people will turn to the new ***SI scientist*** without being afraid of the stigma associated with therapy or social assistance. This field can become a uniquely credible discipline *par excellence* within the academic framework of Information Studies and Librarianship.

Every new academic discipline attracts people from the periphery of the field who wish to develop their skills independently. This is easily done in the framework of Information Science. Information can be sold from home by communication with various data bases. Since this new science is a sensitive field, ***SI scientists*** should be issued with special licenses only after receiving their MA degrees in the specialized field of Social Information.

What Type of Training will the Future *SI Scientist* Undergo?

The development of the field will bring new innovations and training methods in its wake, but the basic lines can be presented here. It should be kept in mind that we are referring to a new discipline composed of different components of technological, humanistic, and social fields. The students need first to be trained in all the existing technological techniques for the retrieval, organization, and processing of information, that is, they need a basic knowledge of hardware and software, and of communication systems, such as Internet and BitNet. They must gain proficiency in information retrieval using both ordinary and original retrieving techniques. The future ***SI scientists*** should be familiar with most of the reference books, information sources, and data bases dealing with the subject of public aid, and should learn how to use the most advanced systems – including hypertext, multimedia, and artificial intelligence.

In addition, they must have a basic knowledge in managing projects, marketing and advertising. They should be aware that they have to keep up with the latest technological innovations by participating in the "continuing education" and special updating services.

So much for the technological-library aspect, but what about the social aspect. Students should have a BA degree in one of the social sciences and, in addition, they should take basic courses in fields in which they have no background, such as psychology, social work and social rights, as well as an introduction to medicine, i.e., health care and aid services. In addition to acquiring a sound knowledge of the conventional health services, they should also familiarize themselves with alternative medicine and other therapeutic methods. They should understand the foundations of bibliotherapy by taking basic courses in bibliotherapeutic analysis of literature for children, youth, adults, and the elderly. With regard to bibliotherapy, they should also be introduced to the art of story-telling and group dynamics. In order to integrate all these different disciplines, there should be introductory and advanced courses on the following subjects: "How to provide Social Information," "The role of the ***SI scientist*** in modern society" and "Assessment of social needs." These courses will deal with the significance and range of the new discipline, such as the role of the ***SI scientist***, the practical application of the various different skills, the information needs of the public, and the boundaries and limitations of the profession. It is also recommended that students learn a seemingly new "profession," that is, "how to give information to those in need."

As I will explain in the following chapters, this is an art in itself, and its main function is to present alternatives to the consumer in a balanced way, with empathy and objectivity. Since this new discipline will have a scientific research base as well as a practical aim, it is also important to teach research methods and statistical analysis, and to develop continuing courses about society's changing needs and advanced technologies. The development of this discipline in the departments for Information Studies and Librarianship will naturally lead to MA and Ph.D. theses, "discussion groups," and many new and creative projects.[1]

What will be the Function of the Future *SI Scientist*?

Following are some of the possible functions of the ***SI scientist***, depending on how the field develops. Each of the functions listed here can exist on its own or in an integrated system, depending on the framework of the ***SI scientist***'s work. First, there is the administrative aspect. The ***SI scientist*** will manage a Social Information Bank or an Information Office either within a public library, in a community center, or in a hospital library. He or she will specialize in locating material and adapting it for public use. If the Social Information Bank lacks certain material information, the ***SI scientist*** will have all the necessary skills and tools to locate it. The new ***SI scientists*** will function as the "middlemen" between the information and the public. They will talk with the clients, provide them with appropriate information, help them to understand the information when necessary, and even play an active role by helping them to make contact with individuals, institutions, or organizations. In places without public Social Information Banks, the ***SI scientist*** could set up operations on a smaller scale, such as in self-help sections in public libraries. He or she can reinforce the information and referral services, and help publicize the library's social activities.

Another possible function is the creation of special hospital libraries and Information Centers for patients and their families, and the establishment of an Information and Guidance Center within voluntary aid organizations, such as those for cancer and Aids patients. The ***SI scientist*** can set up Information Centers for preventive medicine in community centers, schools, and public libraries and, in addition, organize Information Centers for social rights. These latter centers would have the task of clarifying the law and the rights of the citizen in the event of social problems, family illness, divorce, death, etc. This would involve the obtaining of basic legal information and the referencing of people to specific individuals or institutions which provide professional counseling. The new ***SI scientist*** can be the driving force in organizing local "book clubs" for special groups, such as senior citizens; the aim of these clubs will be social interaction, enjoyment, and entertainment in an intellectual and supportive environment. The ***SI scientist*** will also have the ability to instruct people in distress on how to link up with an electronic "supportive communication group," which will be especially useful for the handicapped and the homebound elderly. The ***SI scientist*** will be able to organize and develop "volunteer groups" to read books and operate computer and multimedia games, especially for children in hospitals and for the elderly in nursing homes. He or she will also be a "reading counsellor," specializing in choosing books needed by hospital staff and mental health institutions for bibliotherapy sessions. Such a service already exists in several institutions, for example, in the St Elizabeth Hospital in Washington, where it is the librarian's task to locate literature for bibliotherapeutic and bibliodiagnostic purposes.[2]

The ***SI scientist*** can serve as adviser to private projects or government offices dealing with welfare and social projects; he or she can be the specialist who locates information, and who gives advice on organization, and on how to make the information more easily understood for public consumption, and can also be consulted, as the recognized expert in the field for the marketing of social projects.

In which Frameworks will the *SI Scientist* Work?

In the first instance, the ***SI scientist*** will work in a public framework where there is a demand for understanding and awareness of the interaction between information and social need: e.g., health, welfare, and judicial government offices. The ***SI scientist*** can work in hospitals, rehabilitation centers, nursing homes, outpatient clinics, as well as schools and public libraries. The ***SI scientist*** can be a consultant for organizations involved with specific illnesses, and international aid organizations such as the Red Cross. It is possible that the certified ***SI scientist*** will work from home as a private agent (with a formal government license), providing a broad spectrum of services in the areas of health, aid, and welfare. They will have all the necessary technology at their fingertips: a computer, modem, and printer, and will also have an expert knowledge of information retrieval. They can act as information advisers to "support groups" and "voluntary organizations" which lack information. A talented and government-licensed ***SI scientist*** will be able to open a Social Information Bank, or act in such a Bank as a government employee.[3]

What are the Boundaries and Limitations of the New Profession?

Because this new profession treads on sensitive ground, and since misleading information or inappropriate reading matter can cause potential damage, limits will have to be set by defining the boundaries of the profession and by issuing a special license for this kind of work, in addition to the required master's degree. First, the ***SI scientists*** must always bear in mind that they are not therapists. Their job is to be mediators, often consulting with other professionals such as physicians, psychologists, social workers, and educational counsellors in the course of their work.

The establishment of each new service should be accompanied by consultations with professionals, and government supervision will be necessary for the creation of local or city Information Banks. The ***SI scientist*** should be certified and the Social Information Bank will become officially recognized and licensed. Every Central Bank should have a board of qualified advisers and specialists who can be called upon to support and help in complicated questions and situations. If the local or federal government takes the initiative in the establishment of an official Information Bank, it will be possible for authorized supervisory committees of experts to be set up. When it is a matter of small projects, such as "book clubs" in community centers, public libraries, or libraries for patients in nursing homes and hospitals, it is advisable for there to be a local advisory board of experts available to give assistance or make decisions when problems arise.

It is possible that most of the problems will arise in the private sector, where the ***SI scientist*** acts independently and there is no way to be sure of the quality and reliability of this individual's work in advance. For this purpose a government body should be set up for the granting of licenses to set up private Information Centers; these licenses would be granted according to the suitability of the character and knowledge of the candidate. Issue of the license would be conditional on the candidate holding an MA degree, passing special personality and credibility tests, and having the guaranteed support of two counsellors whenever necessary. A certificate attesting to his or her membership in a professional organization for Social Information scientists would be sine qua non. This organization would be there to provide help and supervision as needed. Another function of the SI professional organization would be to determine a reasonable price for the sale of social information so that the consumer would not be overcharged. The precise definition of the ***SI scientist***'s work would have to be anchored in the law, and the boundaries of the job clearly delineated: to organize and establish Information Banks; to assist people in finding institutions, organizations, and social activities; to provide bibliographical services through the recommendation of scientific literature, reference books, literary works, and other kinds of media. The ***SI scientist*** would be formally obligated to protect the privacy of clients and, at the same time, this individual should also be protected against spurious legal claims. The citizen receiving information services from a public organization or from a Social Information scientist would be required to sign a short document confirming the receipt of information, not professional counseling, and that he or she alone has the right to choose how that information should be used.[4]

The final, but no less important, question is: will we really need a middleman in an advanced technological world in which every person will have his or her own home computer and means of communication. The answer is an unequivocal, yes. There is no comparison between information for purposes of assistance, and simple, direct information such as show schedules, listings of store opening hours, ordering from the supermarket via computer, and buying stocks from the stock exchange. We are talking here about a completely different category of information.

The whole subject of locating information for people in distress is complicated, and is often related to situations of stress, fear, and helplessness. Will the private citizens, unaware of important, concealed sources of information and of the strategies of information retrieval, be capable of locating the information they need by themselves when in a state of emotional crisis?

Let us take the relatively simple example of an old man who has been hospitalized by his son in a nursing home: if his son attempts to locate information on nursing institutions on his own, he will receive an almost endless list, but may not be aware that additional data are available which provide all the necessary details, from the cost to a description of services offered, as well as names of voluntary organizations that can help him. Merely striking a key on the computer is not enough. He will not know that there is a book that describes his father's problem and its influence on the family. I doubt that it will even occur to him at this time to look for a support group for himself or any other member of the family. In other words, although he is capable of finding a lot of information by himself, he probably would not have the skills to select and classify it to his best interest. It seems unlikely that people in stressful situations are capable of sorting through data, conducting on-line searches, and selecting the most appropriate choices from the vast amounts of material available.

Most perceptive people are probably able to analyze their problems and find partial answers, but even they need support and a friendly shoulder during difficult times. In order for our society to have a large group of people able to understand what information is and its vast potential and limitations, Social Information should be taught as part of the compulsory curriculum for the new generation of young people. When this generation grows up, the need for the ***SI scientist***'s services will diminish and change, but that is a long way ahead . . .

7

Establishing the New Discipline

In this chapter I present a possible scenario of the future practical applications in the field of Social Information Science. A basic outline of projects, both new and ongoing, is sketched. This outline, after further refinement, needs to be brought to the public's attention. The following can serve as a pioneering guide.

Once governments become aware of the enormous potential of the 21st century's most important resource, tremendous progress can be achieved. Government involvement can bring about the proper institutionalization of the discipline; it can legitimize the new profession and heighten public awareness. Government intervention will also facilitate the creation of an international aid communications network for specialists and laymen alike. In any case, with or without this government involvement, the already existing awareness and knowledge will stimulate the creation of original projects. Once departments for Information Studies and Librarianship recognize the discipline and educate skilled professionals to serve as *SI scientists*, social welfare will have taken a giant step forward.

There are many practical applications that can be developed in order to increase welfare and health. Here are six main applications:

I Establishing formal Social Information Banks – SI Banks
II Adapting and editing direct information
III Adapting and editing literary works, poetry, and films
IV Developing and adapting advanced electronic technologies
V Developing community projects

VI Developing national and international projects.

I. Establishing Formal Social Information Banks

(1) Social and Health Information Centers

The function of Social and Health Information centers will be to provide the public with basic information on social problems and health issues. They would be established nationwide as municipal or local centers that operated either as independent establishments or as part of public libraries or community centers. The client would receive a list of relevant institutions and organizations; he or she could then consider social assistance and medical options, and become acquainted with research literature, basic legal books as well as literary works, films, and cassettes – all according to the specific needs of the individual. The man or woman in the street would leave the center with a tool: a name, address, phone number, or book. He or she would also leave the center with several alternatives, with enough information to determine which solution was the most appropriate. In this way individuals will learn how to cope with their problems more effectively; they will know how to identify the problem and its physical and social side effects. They will know that they are not alone in coping with such a problem, that there is more than one possible solution, and even if there is no solution, they will still be able to choose the most suitable course of action. Another advantage of such centers is that the sources of information are all to be found under one roof so that one does not have to go from place to place in order to gather information. The person leaving such a center with a computer printout containing addresses, a reference book, or a story similar to his or her own, will be much surer of himself or herself than the individual who is helplessly wondering how to deal with a problem. Electronic communication by telephone, fax, or E-mail will of course enable people to make contact with the Center without leaving their homes.

The name given to this institution is very significant. In effect,

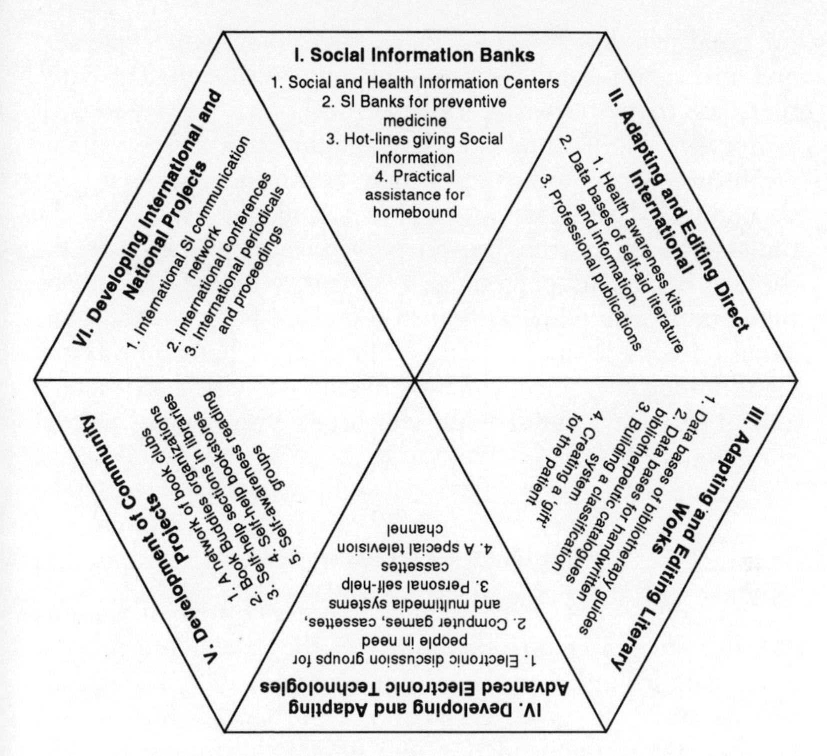

The Spectrum of Social Information Science Activities

we already have small information centers, set up in government social offices, and referral services in public libraries. But in order to adopt "aid through information" into the human ecological and social well-being of the next century, it is advisable that these institutions operate on a different basis, and have a special new name – Social Information Banks, or, in short, SI Banks.

(2) SI Banks for Preventive Medicine

In addition to the social services that the SI Bank can provide, it can also be used for educational projects, such as increasing the awareness of preventive medicine. Information can be provided on the prevention of illnesses and the basic requirements for good health, good nutrition, giving up smoking, safe sex, and protection from harmful elements. Although, currently, there are many television advertisements on these subjects, it is not enough. Printed booklets should always be available for browsing. While it is true that we are advancing toward becoming a "paperless society," it is still important that the publication of information on preventive medicine be in the form of books and pamphlets, so that they can be used at any time and in any place without too much effort. These centers should become a routine part of 21st-century human tradition. Children can be trained while still in school to visit these centers; and in this way, the SI Bank will become an integral part of community life.[1]

(3) Hot-Lines – Emotional First Aid

Most countries now offer telephone services for emotional first aid, but after talking to the volunteer the person still remains alone with his or her problem. Whenever possible, this first-aid service could be given through the SI Bank, which would combine the recommendation of a suitable institution with the suggestion of appropriate literature. In this way, the individual hanging up the phone would no longer be alone, but would be faced with the task of getting up in the morning, and going out to get the appropriate information or a book that would enable that person to identify with a particular character. This, of course, will not work in every case, and may not be practical or successful, but the very fact of the person in distress knowing that he or she has an address – the SI Bank – where advice can be obtained, is already a giant step forward in cultivating self-confidence and a constructive approach for people in need.[2]

(4) Practical Assistance for the Homebound

The SI Bank can provide practical help for homebound disabled people, such as arranging the delivery of medical supplies, sending volunteers to help during an emergency situation, and shopping for food. This project can operate either as a branch of the SI Bank or as a separate entity. This branch will actively offer practical assistance. It will be a service not for actual medical emergencies, when an ambulance should be called (though the center might also serve as a communication center with the hospital), but rather, for seemingly simple situations that are, nevertheless, of importance to the patient. A temporary lack of food supplies, a technical problem, an urgent need for help in a certain activity – all these are potential emergencies for the disabled. The sense of security that contact with such a center provides would be most valuable.

II. Adapting and Editing Direct Information

(1) Health-Awareness Kits Recorded on Audio, Video, CD-Rom

The creation of "health kits" will be a source of relevant information on disease and preventive medicine. Such literature and cassettes can already be found today in the health sections of book stores. Since we are aiming for a broad aid program, it is advisable that the information contained in these books and cassettes be accurate, reliable, and based on academic research. Just as various products carry labels indicating the manufacturer and the fact that the product has undergone quality control, so these health kits should have a label attesting to their quality. It is proposed that a department in the Ministry of Health or Welfare be responsible for the examination of these "products." These kits could be sold in bookstores, in SI Banks, and could also be loaned from public libraries or through the communications network, such as the Internet. They would provide help for patients who are ignorant about their disease, its development, and methods of treatment. The kits should be scientific, reliable, easy to understand, and inexpensive. The contents should include recommendations as to where additional information can be obtained. Health kits could, of course, be developed for most kinds of social problems – divorce problems, for example, where information could be provided on marriage counselors, family therapists, and even basic legal information. With our advanced technology, many diverse and sophisticated kits could be devised using a combination of windows and imaging techniques. It is even possible that a small multimedia system could be designed that, in addition to the information mentioned, would allow an interview with a physician or other specialist. These health and social kits could be developed with the help of the *SI scientist* and social experts to comprise most of the different systems available: combining advanced technology with mental/physical and health knowledge.

(2) Building Scientific Data Bases on the Subject of "Self-aid Literature and Information"

Studies dealing with the possible connection between self-help information and literature are found in most social science fields: psychology, sociology, preventive medicine, criminology, education, librarianship, etc. Their consolidation into a unified research data base will allow us to be exposed to most of the existing material. In addition to theoretical studies, these data bases should also include ongoing research projects and practical applications. This will enable a heightening of the alertness of the academic world to the potential of social information, resulting in new scientific theories and practical programs. It is also important to open the way for a permanent electronic discussion group for specialists, *SI scientists*, and high-tech producers. Such a "discussion group" would lead to a constant flow of ideas and creativity, thus causing the discipline to flourish.

(3) Publication of Academic Research

As in any academic discipline, this new field of Social Information will require a recognized outlet for publication, such as journals dealing with "information and society," "social needs and advanced technology," etc. It is also important to hold national and international conferences, and to publish the proceedings.

III. Adapting/Editing Literature, Poetry, Films

As pointed out earlier, the field of bibliotherapy is mindful of the use of literary elements as a source of aid. While the use of information as a source of aid is direct, literature is sometimes used indirectly for emotional needs such as self-awareness, identity, catharsis, and a better understanding of reality. The adapting of direct information is relatively easy, since data can be classified according to social needs. The creation of a method to classify literature is much more difficult, since everyone finds a different personal inner world in a book that cannot be known to the person editing and classifying the material. In order to understand this point, I quote the Russian scholar Nicholas Rubakin (1862–1946):

> A book, as a material object, will be differently perceived by different people. In our view, when the book is being read it is a subjective psychological phenomenon based on impressions which the reader's psycho-physical organism receives from it as an external object. Should the reader's organism undergo some change (through illness, ageing, etc.) the same book would seem very different to him. Therefore, the book in itself, as a phenomenon independent of the viewer, is an unknown entity . . . The reader does not attribute the psychological phenomena evoked by a text to himself; he attributes them to the book, which is a material object. He objectifies them and projects them onto the book . . . [3]

Despite this limitation, there have been several attempts to classify literary material from a bibliotherapeutical point of view. Most of these attempts use very basic direct methods, focusing on the main topic of the book. Despite the difficulties, it is possible to develop other, more sophisticated methods of classification and to conduct relevant projects. It is important to emphasize that, from the quantitative point of view, the approach to the literature's subject matter should be different from the approach to direct information. It is possible to conduct bibliotherapeutical activities using a relatively small number of books in rehabilitation centers, hospitals and even in social clubs. An organized list of 50–150 books is quite sufficient – initially, at least, it is not necessary to include all pertinent literature. This is in contrast to the field of direct information, in which every shred of information is important: name, telephone number, address, etc. Regarding literature, poetry, and films, the most important thing initially is the quality of the composition, its classification, and its suitability for the consumer. What are the main applications in which literary works can be used as a means for help and support?

(1) Building Data Bases of "Bibliotherapy Guides"

There is currently a considerable number of bibliotherapy guides which have been classified using basic methods, for example, *Reflections – A Subject Guide to Fiction and Biography on Illness and Disability*, by R. B. Tabor and J. Stephenson (1989); and *Bibliotherapy Discussion Group Newsletter*, published by the American Library Association, which has regularly published recommended lists for libraries. The listing of such guides can be found in the basic bibliotherapeutic literature. The material in each of these guides has been classified differently, but the fact of their compilation is important for the creation of a basic "bibliotherapy data base." Important material can also be found in the marginal comments of research studies in the fields of literature, education, and bibliotherapy, recommending relevant reading matter. It would be a good idea, perhaps, to create a special citation index for these studies.[4]

(2) Data Bases for "Handwritten Bibliotherapy Catalogs"

Over the last few years handwritten catalog cards have been compiled by librarians in centers involved in bibliotherapy, such as the St Elizabeth Hospital, the library of the Children's Clinic in the University Hospital in Munich, and various other hospital libraries. Even if its classification is not unified, it is important that this material be concentrated and processed by electronic means. A lot of thought and effort has been invested in these catalogs and the study of their different philosophies of classification would be rewarding.

(3) Building a Classification System

As mentioned above, it is difficult to know which book suits which problem because of the many factors that have to be taken into account: the patient's reading level, knowledge of languages, age, mental state and his or her inner world and mood. I would like to propose an indirect method of classification which does not provide clear and direct solutions, but does contain enough data to give the professionals (e.g. the bibliotherapists, the ***SI scientists***) – and even individual readers – access to the appropriate literature. I do not mean the choosing of a certain book for a particular person or group, but rather, the presentation of a very general approach which can provide us with an initial means of coping with a problem.[5]

I suggest the compilation of a data questionnaire for each book, movie, or poem. This questionnaire would include ordinary bibliographical details and additional details describing the book, for example:

(A) Bibliographical details: name of author, title of book, publisher, place and year of publication.
(B) Is the book listed in a bibliotherapy index or guide?
(C) The content of the literary work:
 1 Main topics
 2 Literary form (prose, poetry, etc.)
 3 Summary of the plot
 4 The main heroes
 5 Setting (place, village, city, room, institution)
 6 How the hero or heroine copes
 7 Solutions hinted at
 8 Style
 9 Suitability for particular age group
 10 Graphic and/or audio-visual means.

When a significant number of such questionnaires have been collected, representing a reasonable number of books, we can then begin to classify the books using such technological methods as hypertext and "windows," thus enabling broader access than that provided by the direct classification system. Let us take the example of a boy hospitalized with cancer; it is doubtful that he will be interested in reading about cancer, it is more likely that he needs to be distracted and entertained. After thorough investigation, it is learned that his main hobby is reading about spaceships and astronauts. By searching for the above items through the computerized questionnaire, it should be easy to find suitable material. When a more complex therapeutic process is required, such as coping with problems in personal relationships, the hypertext method, which enables the finding of all kinds of links, may be more suitable. Through the hypertext search in the questionnaire, it will be possible to obtain the name of the most suitable book, but the decision on whether this item should be used or not must be left to the therapeutic specialist. It is important to try and build up a uniform national or international approach, leading to the creation of basic bibliotherapy data bases for use by hospitals, community centers, and therapists all over the world. This system will also be beneficial for laymen using literature for self-analysis. Again, it must be stressed that I am referring only to the initial classification. Bibliotherapy is a very sensitive field since it involves the human soul, and along with the use of computerized systems, it is recommended that a specialist be consulted.[6]

(4) A Gift for the Patient – Or a Gift for the Promotion of Well-being and Health

One of bibliotherapy's characteristics is the creation of a situation where a distressed person can identify with a book hero, and thus learn a positive and productive approach which, hopefully, will help this individual to live a more constructive life. Not every person, however, can be expected to read lengthy biographies. People who enjoy reading or those involved in lengthy sessions of psychotherapy can do it easily, but how can we help the majority of people needing advice, who have neither the time, training, will, nor the experience to enter an extensive reading process?[7]

There is a solution for such people which is both novel and fresh in approach. Weekly and daily newspapers, popular journals, and literary magazines contain a great deal of biographical material, a fascinating documentation of people who live among us – including some who have undergone difficult experiences such as diseases, accidents, or the loss of loved ones. These articles are easy to read; as they are about our contemporaries, they are also convincing. If all these articles were to be categorized and published in booklet form, the ***SI scientists*** working in hospitals, rehabilitation centers, nursing homes, community centers, etc. could refer patients to the appropriate biographical booklets. Today, using advanced multimedia techniques, it is already possible to create an electronic book that, using "windows" techniques, can even include a live interview with the subject of the biography. Being able to see the speaker's face, movements and vitality will have a great effect on those coping with similar problems. Such electronic material can also be used at home and in health institution discussion groups. Another possible therapeutic element that can be included in this treatment is a special cassette containing exercises for relaxation, positive thinking, and guided imagination.

One of the innovations of the 20th century is the discipline of psychoneuroimmunology, which has been used in cancer clinics such as the Simonton Clinic in Dallas, Texas. This discipline has shown that positive thought and guided imagination exercises can enhance the physical rehabilitation process. The person in crisis has read the book/booklet, and seen and heard the hero or heroine on the television or computer screen; the patient should now be provided with a tool to help him or her continue the effort to develop a positive approach. This tool could be a cassette promoting relaxation and positive thought, and might contain instructions for imagination exercises, where the "known hero" is mentioned, and the patient is then instructed to try to "enter" into this positive and healthy character. For example, a cancer patient undergoing exhausting chemotherapy treatment and trying to cope with the illness may derive encouragement from reading a booklet about a person who has been through a similar experience, recounting their feelings during treatment and subsequent cure. A cassette about positive thinking, instructing a person on how to relax and to imagine stepping into the character of a hero or heroine, will promote inner strength and encourage the healing process.

The publishing of biographical booklets and the production of self-help cassettes could become a very lucrative business, particularly if such items become common and acceptable presents for sick people and people in distress in the coming century. These relaxation cassettes and the choice of literary texts for the booklets need to be made not by publishers alone, but in coordination with experts in the therapeutic field. As in bibliotherapy sessions, here, too, experts should be consulted in the choice of the right booklet or cassette for each individual case. A similar concept can be applied to films – a movie with a positive and productive message can encourage the patient and lift his or her spirits, while a comedy will be relaxing and provide a distraction.[8]

IV. Developing and Adapting Advanced Electronic Technologies

The information available to us today is found in various different technological forms that can be used in order to help people. We can use the older forms of printing, audio and video, and also the modern data bases and computer software, electronic publications, compact disks and multimedia systems which combine all the techniques. Just the fact that now, as we approach the 21st century, we have so many different ways of processing information, allows us to think of unique new projects for the benefit of society. In the previous section I gave an example of how the sick could benefit. Some major achievements have been made in the 20th century, such as the use of Braille and talking books for the blind, and other adaptive technologies. There is a broad range of possibilities for developing the new discipline, some of which are presented below.

(1) Electronic Discussion Groups for People in Need

The use of electronic mail (E-mail) is increasing. There are communication networks today through which researchers from all parts of the world can exchange ideas. The formation of such a group of "friends," dealing with a common problem and wanting to share their experiences with people in the same situation, can lead to the establishment of a communications network – for this purpose all that is needed is a simple PC and a basic knowledge of how it works. The future ***SI scientist***, who will be able to identify the needs of society and the specific groups in society requiring this service, can – within the framework of a job as manager of the SI Bank – help those interested in finding a group of "friends" to be connected to such a group. There are several groups within society whose lives could be changed for the better by such a possibility, for example, those with speech and hearing disorders will be able to "speak" to people using E-mail, and a new world will open up before them. In other cases this group need not necessarily deal with problems; it could also be a kind of "electronic social club."

(2) Computer Games, Cassettes and Multimedia Systems

Computer games have conquered the world over the last few years. Over the past decade, the contest on the screen between good and evil, winner and loser, has become an integral part of social life.[9] These tools can also be used for other applications, of which we must become aware. For example, why shouldn't games be developed around health issues, with a positive message that can be used for the elderly or for sick children? Instead of chasing the bad guy or killer, why not chase after a treasure that will bring good health, happiness, and laughter – the applications are endless. A boy with a poor self-image can enter the persona of Gulliver, a confident, powerful man. The boy will travel great distances over mountains and oceans, lakes and rivers until he reaches Gulliver's home where he will receive a prize: the Golden Ball representing good health, strength, and confidence. At the end of the game, Gulliver will ask the player to imagine that he is holding his Golden Ball at times when he is in need of strength and encouragement. Even though it sounds simplistic, the imaginative use of "Gulliver's Golden Ball," as proved by the new science of psychoneuroimmunology, has great therapeutic value. In another example: a woman lacking confidence will seek a "tool" to help her on her long quest; she reaches the forest, enters the room of treasures, and there is ordered to select one tool from the many to be found there – golden coins, diamonds, books, old scrolls, etc. The player will choose an "imaginative tool," a tool that lifts her inner world, a tool that inspires confidence, and she will be told to imagine using this special tool in times of distress or lack of confidence.[10]

Perhaps one of the reasons that computer games are so popular is because they express our inner need to fight and win. If this is true, why should a game not be developed in which a sick patient can slowly "kill" his illness? We recognize the fact that people in distress need someone to talk to or to believe in. Some people use the church, synagogue, or mosque; others use friends. Others, unable to cope, use drugs. Why not teach people through these "games" that there is "someone in their own mind" who can always be with them, and that this "someone" can be shaped in any form that is convenient or familiar to them. Of course, this is only one of many applications, and these games should only be used after appropriate instruction. Such games in hospitals or other health institutions could contribute a great deal to the confidence and positive thinking of the patients. Why not use our sophisticated advanced technology to encourage positive thinking and self-esteem? Even the skeptics among us need something positive and secure to hold on to during a crisis; even if it isn't a complete cure, it still provides support and indirectly helps the body to come to terms with the problem and, sometimes, even to heal itself.

(3) Personal Self-help Cassettes

A tremendous number of self-help cassettes already exist: cassettes related to relaxation, proper diet, pregnancy, overcoming depression, building self-confidence, and so on. All of these cassettes have one thing in common: they are designed for a large group of people who share a problem. The cassettes are not meant to fulfill each individual person's specific needs. Today, as we understand more about the function of the brain and thought processes, there is no doubt that these cassettes can arouse positive and constructive forces in the body. It is true that they cannot provide a total solution to a problem, nor are they a substitute for psychological or medical treatment, but they do have a salutary foundation that has a calming effect on people and leads them in a positive direction. In order to increase the efficiency of such cassettes, I suggest expanding the field and developing special personalized cassettes. This service can be carried out in SI Banks, or in the social service offices or hospitals, either in coordination with the ***SI scientists***, or with the guidance of a suitable expert. The intention here is to use all the existing techniques and integrate them into programs suited to a particular person. For example: nineteen-year-old Dorothy has a weight problem; a personalized cassette can be prepared for her. It will include relaxation and imaging exercises, as well as comments relating to her personal and specific personality. The person preparing the cassette should be an expert from the field of therapy, and should ask Dorothy several basic questions when preparing the cassette, such as: which non-fattening foods do you like? Dorothy's answer might be – cold lemonade. Another question could be: at what hours do you tend to overeat? The answer –

between 6 p.m. and 7 p.m. These elements can then be incorporated into personalized cassettes in the following ways. First, Dorothy's first name will be mentioned: instead of the words "Heal yourself," the cassette will use the words, "Dorothy, heal yourself." Instead of "You are in a safe and quiet place" – "Dorothy, you are in a safe and quiet place." The details provided by the patient will be incorporated: "Dorothy, every time you drink cold lemonade, your condition will improve, your body will become more beautiful and more attractive. Every evening between 6 and 7 you will feel calm, happy, and safe . . . , etc." I have purposely refrained from using the words "weight gain" or "loss," since focusing on the problem only makes it worse, as Émile Coué, one of the founding fathers of autosuggestion, stated at the beginning of the 20th century.

Another situation in which a personalized cassette can be significant is in the case of a patient who is unconscious or in a coma. It is known that in such conditions, people can sometimes absorb and understand what they hear, but cannot react. There are many stories about relatives who sit for hours at the patient's bedside talking to him or her. In such a case it is best to prepare a very personal cassette, with details of the patient's life, hobbies, and favorite music. Such cassettes can also be used with anesthetized patients during surgery. How effective is such a cassette? It varies from person to person. It cannot be expected to solve the problem, but it does make it a little easier for relatives who want to do everything possible for their loved one. The technological preparation of such cassettes is relatively easy; all that is required is a recording studio and a person qualified in guided imagination, who has a knowledge of the patient's personality. Such cassettes can also be prepared for people going into surgery. The text can be organized by the patient prior to the operation, and will be used during and after surgery – this will have a favorable impact on the patient's recovery, will promote the feeling that the patient is in control, and allow the person to take an active part in his or her own recovery.[11]

(4) A Special Television Channel for Social Information

The subject of health and welfare is dealt with on many television networks throughout the world – from morning exercises to the latest medical information and interviews with specialists and patients.

Why launch a special channel for "social information" and not settle for the standard programs? Because the constant existence of a specially designated channel can create a "support group" for millions of people around the world. We all need help at certain times in our lives. The existence of such a channel would take the secrecy out of problems that people are loath to discuss. In the 21st century people will be aware that such problems are an integral part of life, that there is no need to hide or isolate oneself, and that problems can be coped with and sometimes even used constructively. A special television channel, set up with the help of qualified experts, will enable the population of the world to receive a wide range of information and to learn methods for coping. What should this channel include? The first thing that comes to mind is a program of exercises (as well as an exercise program for the physically disabled, which can be performed sitting or lying down). The network should include programs with relaxation and guided imagination exercises. It could also include comedy films, movies with a positive and constructive message, and "laughter exercises." It should also provide information on the power of faith and positive thought, together with information on the latest conventional health care. The network will bring to the public's attention the fact that people have a choice, and, in many cases, an alternative to what they already know. There will be interviews with people who have overcome crises, emphasizing their methods of coping and their accomplishments. In addition, the network will give information about the existence of SI Banks, books, cassettes, rehabilitation and aid programs, volunteer organizations, and so on. There is a further possibility of the network organizing a "bibliotherapy program" based on a movie or a poem, just like the story-teller of old. The individual in distress will know that at any hour of the day or night, advice, information and guidance can be found, as well as relaxation sessions and entertainment, on the special SI channel.[12]

V. Developing Community Projects

Interesting projects can be developed around the central theme of support information and literature even within small communities.

(1) A Network of "Book Clubs"

Although it is possible that books might disappear altogether in the coming era, their content can still be used in the new electronic or in the old printed form. "Community book clubs," whose members include teenagers, adults, the elderly, or combined groups, will meet to discuss the content of a particular book, poem, or film. A joint discussion about a book, though not formally connected to the members' everyday problems or exposing them, may nevertheless act as a beneficial tool for releasing tensions, for incidental conversations about problems, and for obtaining knowledge on the reactions of other people to problems and crises. For anyone interested in getting out of the framework of the house, the television and the computer, this will be a social solution as well as an opportunity to open up and expose oneself to new subjects, alternatives, and novel approaches. The *SI scientists* in the SI Banks will organize these clubs. The organizer may invite a known writer, or a health/welfare professional. The meetings can be led by the *SI scientist*, who will be trained in group dynamics. The main idea here is not therapy, but rather, "social interaction" and the exchange of opinions and ideas. Such activity unofficially takes place today in the framework of the public libraries, but it is still difficult to turn the public library into a social club. In contrast, regular meetings in relatives' homes or in the framework of the formal community center can help improve the social atmosphere. In this way, the "printed book" will take on a new image as a tool for social interaction, a tool to alleviate the "solitariness" of the computer age.

(2) "Book Buddies" Organizations

A "Book Buddy" is someone who reads books to people in distress, usually on a voluntary basis. As mentioned earlier, this activity was initiated in San Francisco, where the public library developed an impressive project, and trained volunteer "Book Buddies" to read to patients in local hospitals. The "Book Buddies" wear a special badge, carry a special bag, and read to children using special props such as dolls and crayons. The main aim of this project is not the actual reading but, rather, the personal supportive bond. This bond is reminiscent of the "story-telling" of the pre-television era and even of pre-printing days, when villagers or family members sat down in the evenings and listened to stories told by their elders.

The flourishing of the art of "story-telling" proves that even today, in this computerized and advanced era, man and woman have strong desires for stories and the emotions they arouse. Projects such as "Book Buddies" can develop in different frameworks, and can employ different methods: they can be carried out in nursing and rehabilitation institutions, and in community centers. They can also act as a kind of mobile book club, in which a reader comes to the home of the elderly, the lonely, or the disabled. Volunteers can be of any age, and there is no doubt that they will find it as rewarding as their listeners.

(3) Self-help Sections in Libraries

Public libraries contain an enormous amount of literature that is a potential source of assistance. For those seeking information, there are libraries with Information and Referral Services, but only a small proportion of libraries contain a self-help section that includes both literary works and direct information books. Public awareness of the sources of help to be found in public libraries must be heightened so that people will know how to use these important establishments for social needs. Another idea would be to open self-help sections in school libraries, where there are many young people with problems. It is important to give such a section an appropriate name, since the concept of "self-help" might scare people away, among other reasons, out of fear of invasion of privacy. It could be called "the self-awareness section" of the SI Bank.[13]

(4) Self-help Bookstores

There are many bookstores nowadays that specialize in alternative medicine, mysticism, astrology, fortune-telling, etc. The existence of these stores testifies to the public need for this service. There should be bookstores representing the entire spectrum of health and aid – both conventional and unconventional – and selling books in both electronic and printed form. The clientele of these stores will be those who do not wish to go to public institutions for information, or people wanting to expand their knowledge on certain subjects. The certified *SI scientist* might well work in such a store as a consultant, helping customers choose books.

(5) Self-awareness Reading Groups

Joseph Gold, the author of *Read for your Life* (1990), explains the important spiritual contribution made by literature as an integral part of satisfying human needs not otherwise easily appeased, such as anger, violence, the desire for happiness, etc. In his book, Gold shows the reader how to analyze personal reading tastes in order to reveal previously unknown details. In this way the reader becomes more aware of likes and dislikes, what is important and what isn't, to which characters he or she is attracted – and why.[14] We live in a world in which certain sections of the human race are constantly seeking their own identity: leisure time, disappointment with religious institutions, exposure to a tremendous wave of media and information – all contribute to the need to seek understanding and happiness.

Many turn to mystic cults, to old–new healing methods, and others turn to drugs. Another way to seek one's identity is through reading. Small self-awareness reading groups of people searching for themselves, and with the time and will to do it, could also exist in the framework of "book discussion groups" of the SI Bank. In contrast to the "book clubs" mentioned above, which would be directed toward society in general, their purpose being social-entertainment, the self-awareness reading centers would be made up of special groups of people who were ready to put some time into analyzing their own personalities. It would be possible to learn in these centers how to make a personal analysis of reading characteristics, how to learn from those characteristics, and to have open-minded, interesting, enriching discussions. This institution would probably not be as popular as the mystic cults, since it would not boast any magic solutions. The individual turning to a self-awareness group should be prepared to take responsibility for his or her life. A ready-made solution will not be found in these centers, but individuals must seek their own personal solutions through profound personal self-awareness, and not through ignorance and confusion.

VI. Developing National and International Projects

Once the new field of social information gains academic recognition, it will be a lot easier for governments, universities, and SI Banks in various countries to develop international and national projects. Advanced technology will facilitate the creation of a large SI communication network, and all the institutions (including hospitals), projects, and research studies on Social Information will thus become available to people in different parts of the world. Only time will tell if an "international SI network" will develop, but there is no doubt that conducting these projects in many countries will facilitate the establishment of local SI networks within the countries involved. An effort should be made to promote the subject because of its great importance to the human race. The European Community and international organizations such as the UN, the Red Cross, UNESCO, should join the effort. In the initial phase, a network of international and national conferences should be set up where the participants could report on their research, their ideas, and ongoing projects. This will be the beginning of international communication in the area of Social Information. In a world with so much strife, so many health problems, economic difficulties, wars, and conflicts, the awareness of Social Information will help balance the human atmosphere on the side of support, health, peace, and tranquility. Cooperation in support and aid projects can also be a common denominator between rival nations and different religious centers in the world. The common factor of relief, health, and peace can be achieved even in situations of strife and war. Even during periods of hostile conflicts, it should still be possible to set up a network of cooperation and mutual trust by shifting some of the efforts to a common and positive cause. The subject of Social Information can be a basis for productive negotiations, for cooperation and for dialogue. It can serve as a "Bridge between Nations" – a bridge that we all need in order to make our fragile, unstable world a better place to live in.

Byproducts

In this book I have described the benefit that can be gained by people with social and health problems using human knowledge in a positive and creative way. In addition, along with this major achievement, there are also original and unique byproducts in several other fields; first, a new profession will be created in a world full of unemployment – that of ***SI scientist.*** New jobs will also be created in its wake: technology experts and mental health specialists; the publishing world will develop new enterprises and new jobs will thus be created in that area as well. The creation of new projects will increase the number of employees. I am referring not to work initiated specifically in order to solve the problem of unemployment, but rather to a constructive and productive new line of work.

The creation of these new jobs will not be based on government investment, but on the prices the citizens will be charged for these new services.[15] The development of a Social Information field will also partially solve the problems of the elderly. As the quality of life and health care improves, there will be a growing population of senior citizens. Those senior citizens who are able can work – either as volunteers or for token pay – as Book Buddies, managers of book clubs, or assistants in SI Banks. This will be beneficial not only to those in need, but also to the elderly workers themselves – it will keep them occupied, make them feel useful, and provide them with a motivation and a challenge.[16] Another benefit – the development of creative, community activities based on the use of books and information technologies – will open additional channels for spending leisure time in a positive and constructive manner, to the benefit of people and society.

The theory of building a science of Social Information includes the use of the printed book as an integral part of the information society. The book remains but gets a new image – as a tool for self-awareness. This retaining of the book within the process of the information revolution offers a tremendous advantage. It is known that reading books arouses people's imagination and creative ability, an aspect often missing when one receives processed information such as that from television or computers. By leaving the printed book in the framework of an advanced technological society, we will be able to preserve that most vital process – the human imagination – which is responsible for most of humanity's achievements.

The use of human knowledge for positive enterprises should be a matter of common interest for all religions, races, and nations. Politicians and scientists who grasp this concept will be able to develop research projects and practical applications that will promote tranquility, peace, and cooperation throughout the world.[17]

8

Academic Research, Basic Theories and Questions

In addition to the broad practical applications of Social Information, academic research needs to be developed in order to construct a scientifically sound discipline. The right questions should be asked and acceptable research methods developed.

Much can be learned from the "Livre et Société" school of thought that emerged at the end of the 1950s in France. This branch of study began with the well-known book of Lucien Febvre and Henri Jean Martin, *The Coming of the Book* (original version, Paris, 1958; English translation, London, 1976). As one of the founders of the "Annales New Historian," Febvre, who studied human history in the broadest ways possible, indicated the importance of the sociology and history of communication through print. He and his followers studied the history of the printed book from very original points of view. The book and printing for them is not an isolated phenomenon, but is connected to three major factors: (a) the people who create the book (authors, printers, publishers, and booksellers); (b) the people who read books (scholars, students, and laymen); and (c) the elements that influence and shape the visual appearance of the book and its distribution (social and economic factors, religion, education, and leisure activities). If we add to the social concept of "Livre et Société" the new element of modern high-tech technology, we have a starting point for developing the new Social Information Science, a science which will study all the social angles of the inventions of printing and electronic communication systems, ranging from historical and sociological questions to the creation of practical applications for the benefit of society.[1]

There are various important research possibilities but several basic questions have to be answered before they are embarked upon. The first task is to identify the social needs of the public that can be catered for by the use of human knowledge. This should be done according to defined social parameters such as health problems, social problems, leisure activities, and special helping professions. In addition to these formal parameters, other factors have to be included, such as literary knowledge, computer management knowledge, habits of information-gathering, the emotional state, and economic conditions. If we are familiar with the social needs of the public, suitable data bases can be developed and the tools of the ***SI scientist*** will be more accurate and efficient.

In the framework of Librarianship and Information Science, there is now a trend toward conducting studies on the research needs of scientists in the various fields of knowledge. Studies about consumer needs should be used as a model in order to reveal those needs that can be fulfilled by Information, literature, and electronic technologies.[2]

Another fundamental question is: how should the recommendations of information and literature be carried out? How can we show the consumer that information provides alternatives and not always absolute truths? How can this information be delivered in the most balanced and objective way? In the field of medical research there are differences of opinion about the way the patient and the patient's family should be given information. This is a crucial problem when dealing with social and emotional problems. We need a special method of communication with the information consumer – a method that will give hope and support and will stress that there is always a more creative solution, that research showing statistics and figures is not necessarily an automatic death sentence – every person is a unique case and so are his social and health prognoses.

Information can be either constructive or destructive. Even appropriate information, if given in the wrong way, can be damaging. An academic method for imparting information must, therefore, be created with the help of academic studies related to psychology and sociology, using the knowledge relating to the bond between patient and therapist, body language, and NLP (Neuro Linguistic Programming) methods. The proper use of words with the right body language can contribute a great deal to the positive empathic relationship between the person providing the information and the consumer.[3]

The necessary approach is a humane one that will help to release the patient from a state of panic to a state of balance. If we build sophisticated SI Banks with all the latest electronic means of communication, but leave the field of human relationships undeveloped, consumers will not use this new service and the whole concept of using human knowledge for the benefit of the public will fall apart.

Another question that has to be studied is the cost of such a project. Economic and human elements must here be taken into account. The new discipline will have to be profitable if it hopes to attract qualified personnel. On the other hand, not everyone is able to pay significant amounts for information services. This question must be thoroughly examined, taking into account the cost of investment and the contribution to society. A possible solution is for the consumer to be entitled to Social Information within the framework of health insurance. This question cannot be resolved at present; precise academic studies will have to be conducted in order to arrive at an appropriate scheme enabling all those who want to use these new services to do so.

Another question is that of ethics. Just as there are ethical criteria in the field of medicine, familiar to every doctor who has taken the Hippocratic Oath, so there must be ethical codes in the field of Social Information. The information should be delivered with a warm and humane attitude, and the data should be reliable, accurate, and up-to-date. The consumer should be aware that the information is constantly being updated and that one should always check for new information. It must also be understood that, even in the most sophisticated SI Banks, the ***SI scientist*** can never say: "I have given you all the existing information in the field . . . " Even today, with the use of electronic communication methods, there is still always a certain amount of information that does not appear in the data base. If, for example, we take a major reference tool such as "sociological abstracts," this will contain only a selection of articles on any subject and therefore the information about sociology found in this reference tool is obviously incomplete. This is an academic example, but there is no one alive today who can say "I have found everything ever written and printed on a certain subject." This fact must be made equally clear to the consumer and to the ***SI scientist***, so that the consumer will never feel that he or she has left the SI Bank with "absolute" information, which could lead to great disappointment in extreme cases. The ***SI scientist***'s task is not to formulate decisions, but rather, to facilitate the consumer's access to most of the existing possibilities.

The next question is one usually dealt with in the fields of philosophy and psychology: when the available information is negative, as in the case of severe health problems such as cancer or Aids, how should the information be conveyed? Perhaps – in certain difficult cases – the information should be withheld from the patient? Just as there is film censorship, perhaps in particularly stressful cases there should be information censorship. This is a difficult question and there is no easy solution. At this early stage I can foresee several possible solutions. First, the ***SI scientist*** will not be permitted to "issue a death sentence" – the least that he will be able to say is "according to the information that I have, which appears in such and such sources, . . . most of the people who have had this illness were not cured, but the quality of their lives was significantly improved with the help of medical treatment, proper nutrition, support groups, etc." In other words, a positive and productive attitude should be maintained. This leads us to a major ethical question faced by doctors almost every day: should a patient or his family be told that there is no cure, or should they be left with some hope? Certainly there will be no magical solution to this problem even in the next century. It seems to me, however, that emphasizing the positive, constructive aspects and presenting alternatives is the best possible solution. There is no element here of leading someone on, since miracles do occur every day in the world of medicine and in society. Even if the medical information presents a hopeless picture, why should a dying man lose hope? Even if there really is no absolute answer, the ***SI scientist*** should be aware of the dilemmas involved in such delicate situations.

Another question that has to be resolved is the legal aspect. There are situations in which the ***SI scientist*** could be sued for giving incorrect and outdated information. It should be clear that it is strictly the consumer's decision and choice as to how the information given is to be used. There will certainly be other legal problems. Legal professionals and ***SI scientists*** will have to find solutions and perhaps, eventually, draw up relevant new laws. Additional questions will concern the copyrights of the information sources and the privacy of the consumer. All of these issues will have to be secured within the law. A possible solution is to formulate a contract or an official agreement in which the rights of the consumer and the responsibilities of the ***SI scientist*** are stipulated.[4]

Another problem that merits discussion is whether it is preferable for the new discipline to be largely in private hands or organized by governments? Those dealing with this issue will have to devise ways to ensure that appropriate and up-to-date information is provided in the most sensitive and responsible way. The new discipline will probably be split between government involvement and private initiative. It will be necessary for governments to issue formal licenses for qualified ***SI scientists***, and a code of standards and quality control will have to be set up for Social Information "products," such as multimedia occupational therapy kits, or audio–video kits containing medical or social information. In addition to these particular topics, ongoing projects should be studied and evaluated, and possible ways of improving them should be recommended. Issues such as the activities of the SI Banks, the community book clubs, etc. can be investigated using the regular social scientific research methods, such as questionnaires and models. The findings of these projects would be published in scientific journals, and will pave the way for a productive and creative discipline. In addition to the academic publicity platform of journals, books, and conferences, there will also be a need for platforms dealing with the methods of cataloging and classifying information, and the exposure of all those connected to the discipline to the modern electronic communications technology. Constant contact and cooperation between professionals from the fields of the humanities, social sciences and technology will lead to the development of special programs which cannot yet be predicted. At a later stage, once scientific studies are finally published, it will be worth examining the research results of the SI science in order to see how the field is developing. This can be done by using "bibliometrics" – the analysis of citations in articles – which will allow an assessment of the main researchers in the field, the leading journals, the topics that are being investigated, and those topics which have not yet been dealt with.[5]

A great number of disciplines and skills merge and overlap in this new profession and, as in any new field, there will be many successes and failures along the way. But all along this road, lined as it is with technological, literary, and humane elements, it is important to remember that this is not the development of a sterile science designed for academic testing alone, but rather, a human and practical field *par excellence* in the service of improving the quality of life. The new discipline should develop with love and faith, through the use of balanced, responsible judgment, and good will.

Epilogue: Will we Say "Si"?

From Ancient Legend to Modern Reality

Throughout this book we have discussed information, books, and electronic communications – and their possible contribution to mankind. I shall conclude with a very ancient legend, one of our literary treasures, called "The Library for the Healing of the Soul."

The story takes place in the distant land of nowhere and everywhere, in no time and at all times. It is a story of a ship sailing at night in a stormy sea. Winds, lightning, and thunder make sailing difficult. In the morning light, the captain discovers that he has lost his way. From far away – through the fog – he manages to make out some spots of light, and he steers the ship toward these unidentified beacons. The captain and his passengers reach a small island with a building in the center, which resembles an ancient palace; it is surrounded by an aura of light. The passengers and the captain disembark, approach the building, and see that it is indeed a beautiful palace. They knock at the gate and a smiling man dressed in white, with a long beard, invites them into the magnificent building. A door opens before them, leading into a giant hall full of shelves of books in all languages and on all subjects. In the middle of the room, around a table piled high with books, people wearing various national costumes sit and read. On the left-hand side the curious guests notice a hidden door, inlaid with gold, that is locked and guarded. The puzzled guests ask for an explanation.

The man who admitted them introduces himself as Archimedes, and welcomes them to "The Library for the Healing of the Soul," where there are books for every man, event and situation. The guests exchange glances. "We have heard about libraries for research and libraries for reading, but is there also a library for the soul? Can books cure people?" Archimedes smiles and says, "Would each of you please choose a book, take it with you and, a year from now, come back and tell me how books can cure." The bewildered guests each select a book as asked, and, after being provided with food and drink, go on their way.

A year passed and, for a reason known only to story-tellers, the same group of travelers again sailed on the same boat with the same captain. And once again there were strong winds and storms, and again they found themselves in the enchanted library. Archimedes opened the door with a smile, and, after the visitors entered, he asked them, "Well, can books heal?" Each guest then told his tale. One reported that he had succeeded in making a sick boy smile by reading a funny story to him; a second recounted that by making use of appropriate information he had helped a friend find a solution to a health problem. A third noted that with the help of a collection of tales he had managed to make the lives of his elderly parents more pleasant, and a fourth related that the book he had taken had helped him find a new profession. And so they continued to talk and give an account of all the amazing things that had happened to them. Archimedes smiled quietly, saying, "Now you know how books can heal." The guests again entered the great hall and chose new books. The concealed door on the left-hand side suddenly opened and a distinguished-looking man emerged; he wore a blue silk robe and a golden aura surrounded him. As he approached the guests with a smile, he said pleasantly, "My name is Rafael. I am in charge of 'The Library for the Healing of the Soul.' Now all of you can join our readers around the world, now you too can enjoy our treasure." He then returned to his room and, as the guests slowly left the building, they suddenly noticed that sparkles of light glimmered within their clothes. They looked at each other in wonder, warmth, and understanding. Since then, year after year, day after day, new guests have come to visit this special library. They come, choose books, and emerge with glitters of light on their clothes, a light that accompanies them on their journeys, helping people all over the world.

So ends the legend. The tale begins nowhere and everywhere; in no time and at all times. Will the people of the 22nd century continue to tell this legend about the people of the previous century? Will "The Library for the Healing of the Soul" become an "International Social Information electronic network" for the benefit of humanity? Will we say "Si" and accept the challenge facing us? These questions cannot yet be answered. The only thing that is abundantly clear is that we have a treasure of "human knowledge" in our possession which can be used, developed, and distributed with wisdom and love, to light the way for people in need and to encourage those who hope for a better life.

Appendix

"Information and Society – Facilitative Librarianship" Curriculum for MA degree in the Department of Information Studies and Librarianship, Bar-Ilan University, Israel

This program originated in 1991 in the framework of continuing studies in librarianship for graduate students. In 1993 it became a recognized program within the framework of MA studies and is now an official line of study. The duration of the studies is 2–3 years.

Today the department includes 300 students for BA and MA degrees and has four fields of speciality: Library Organization, Information Science, Research of Rare Books and Manuscripts, and Information and Society – facilitative librarianship.

The aim of the specialization in "Information and Society" is to increase awareness of the use of books and data bases as supportive tools in the community. Great emphasis is placed on the subject of bibliotherapy, since most of the students have backgrounds in the social sciences and education. The main objectives of the studies are to prepare the students (a) to write creative theses with an interdisciplinary approach combining information and librarianship studies, literature, and the social sciences; and (b) to be involved in various lines of work, as follows:

- Working as a bibliotherapy librarian – a specialist who will classify literature from a therapeutic point of view and guide health-care specialists on how to find suitable printed and electronic material for use in therapy.

- The organization of health-care libraries in hospitals, nursing homes, rehabilitation and senior citizen centers.
- The organization of self-help sections in public libraries.
- The organization of social and medical information banks.
- Managing school and public libraries with knowledge and awareness of the social potential found in books and information systems.

This specialty is based on an interdisciplinary approach and is made up of the following components:

1 Basic courses in librarianship and information studies, including the organization and retrieval of information, library computerization, and library and information-center management.
2 Methods of psychological treatment, including methods which stimulate insight and understanding and those which use unconventional methods such as autosuggestion and guided imagery.
3 Study of the therapeutic aspects of literature and information as illustrated by the various types of literature: books, poetry, cassettes, data bases, and movies (bearing in mind different age groups: children, young people, adults, and senior citizens).
4 Studies of the potential applications of the discipline in existing frameworks, such as in schools, public libraries, and nursing and rehabilitation-center libraries; as well as the theoretical possibilities of a breakthrough of the profession into the framework of Social Information science or the directorship of a medical/social information bank.

Students specializing in this program have two options of study: the first requires the writing of a thesis, and the second does not require a thesis. The requirements for the thesis program are 28 weekly hours (credits) and the requirements for the program without a thesis are 37 weekly hours (credits) over 2–3 years.

Out of 50 students accepted into the MA program in 1993,

10 students (20%) chose this specialization. Out of 66 students accepted into the program in 1994, 16 students (24%) chose this specialization. There are a total of 26 students currently (summer 1995) enrolled in this program, the majority of them have chosen not to write a thesis. A few students have begun writing MA theses on the following subjects:

- The library in the "special school" – in light of new innovations in the area of information science and librarianship.
- Bibliotherapy and multimedia.
- Bibliotherapy in public libraries.
- Building a data base for self-help books and manuals.

Most of the students in this program work in libraries or in the educational system as teachers or educational counselors. Some have already begun – in the framework of their work – to develop the subject in projects such as the creation of self-help sections in school and public libraries; the preparation of manual and computerized bibliographical data bases; initiation of bibliotherapy reading sessions in public and school libraries; and initiation of reading sessions for disabled war veterans and senior citizens. To date (summer 1995), the profession of Social Information does not exist in Israel. The purpose of the Bar-Ilan University program at this stage is to train people to build up the discipline within the framework of their places of work, with the aim that as awareness of the subject grows, a new discipline will be created that will make a major contribution to Israeli society – a society under an unusually intense level of social and political pressure.

Courses

The courses marked with an asterisk (*) are required courses for MA students who have chosen to write a thesis.

Introductory courses: 12 credits (for all students in the department). [A course of 60 hours per year (two hours weekly) is considered a two-credit course.]

Name of course	Number of weekly hours (credits)
Preparatory computer course (*)	0
Introduction to computers (*)	2
Research methods and statistics (*)	2
Introduction to reference work (*)	1
Introduction to the reference book in Jewish studies (*)	1
Cataloging methods (*)	1
Classification methods (*)	1
Computer services in libraries (*)	2
On-line data retrieval (*)	2

Specialization: Information and Society – Facilitative Librarianship

Required introductory courses: 6 credits

Introduction to Information science (*)	2
Introduction to psychology (*)	2
Organizational behavior (*)	1
The reading process – its conscious and subconscious foundation (*)	1

Specialization courses: 16 credits

Library services for groups with special social and health needs (*)	1
Management of the special library	1
Medical bibliotherapy in hospitals, nursing homes and rehabilitation centers (*)	1
Management of school libraries	1
Bibliotherapy aspects in adult literature (*)	2
Bibliotherapy for elderly people	1
Bibliotherapy aspects in children's literature (*)	1
Bibliotherapy aspects in poetry (*)	1
Social science data bases	1
Workshop: Tools in social group work (*)	2
Economy and finance data bases	1

Bibliometrics	1
Special aspects of Information studies	1
The building of data bases in medical institutions (*)	1
Elective course	1

Required seminars: 3 credits

Information and society – facilitative librarianship (*)	1
Scientific research in librarianship (*)	1
The school library	1
Building data bases	1
Planning and evaluation in libraries and information centers	1

Notes

The preliminary quotation is from Theodor H. Nelson, "Electronic Publishing and Electronic Literature," in Edward C. Deland (ed.), *Information Technology in Health Science Education* (New York, London: Plenum Press, 1978), p. 213.

1 Technology and Humanitarianism at the Crossroads

1. See F. W. Lancaster, *Toward Paperless Information Systems* (New York: Academic Press, 1978).
2. Many studies have been written on the information revolution and its influence on society. Some of them are: Kevin McGarry, *The Changing Context of Information, An Introductory Analysis*, 2nd edn (London: Library Association Publishing, 1993); P. Laurie, *The Micro Revolution: A Change for the Better or for the Worse?* (New York: Futura Publications, 1980); Peter Large, *The Micro Revolution Revisited* (London: Frances Pinter, 1984); Tom Forester (ed.), *Computers in the Human Context* (Oxford: Basil Blackwell, 1989); Steve Bankes *et al.*, "Harnessing the Information Technologies," *Information Society* 8 (January 1992), pp. 1–59; Alvin Toffler, *Powershift, Knowledge, Wealth and Violence at the Edge of the 21st Century* (New York: Bantam Books, 1990).
3. Alexandra Meir, "The Gutenberg Project," *Bulletin of the Israel Society of Special and Information Centers* 19 (May 1993), pp. 33–35 (Hebrew).
4. Margaret A. Shotton, "The Cost and Benefit of Computer Addiction," *Behaviour & Information Technology* 10 (1991), pp. 219–30; Robert S. Davidson and Page B. Wally, "Computer Fear and Addiction: Analysis, Prevention and Possible Modification," *Journal of Organizational Behavior Management* 6 (1984), pp.

37–51; Margaret A. Shotton, *Computer Addiction? A Study of Computer Dependency* (London: Taylor & Francis, 1989).

5. On the invention of printing and its influence, see Lucien Febvre and Henri Jean Martin, *The Coming of the Book; The Impact of Printing 1450–1800* (London: NLB, 1976); Elizabeth L. Eisenstein, *The Printing Press as an Agent of Change* (Cambridge: Cambridge University Press, 1979).
6. For the dangers of the information revolution, see C. Brod, *Technostress: The Human Cost of the Computer Revolution* (Reading, MA: Addison-Wesley, 1984); D. Howitt and G. Cumberbatch, *Mass Media, Violence and Society* (London: Elek Science, 1975); Gary A. Marx and Sanford Sherizen, "Monitoring on the Job," in Tom Forester (ed.), *Computers in the Human Context* (Oxford: Basil Blackwell, 1989), pp. 397–406; August Bequai, *Technocrimes* (Lexington, MA: Lexington Books, 1987). Information will play an important role in future wars when it may serve as a tool that can either build or destroy. For example, to see how misleading information can control a certain population or army, cf. Alvin and Heidi Toffler, *War and Anti-war; Survival at the Dawn of the 21st Century* (Boston: Little Brown, 1993), chaps 16, 18.
7. For President Clinton's speeches and commentary, see Marc Cooper, "New Horizons: Clinton's Technology Policy and the Project for Information Superhighways," *Bulletin of the Israel Society of Special Libraries and Information Centers* 19 (May 1993), pp. 43–44. On the Internet and Information Superhighway Project, see Al Gore, "Infrastructure for the Global Village," *Scientific American* 265 (Sept. 1991), pp. 150–53; Tracy Laquey and Jeanne C. Ryer, *The Internet Companion, A Beginner's Guide to Global Networking* (Reading, MA: Addison Wesley, 1993); James K. Lee, "Toward the Information Superhighway," *Telecommunication Policy* 17 (Nov. 1993), pp. 631–35; R. D. Lankes, "National Net 1993 Conference Explores Information Superhighway under Clinton Administration," *Library Hi Tech News* 104 (July–August 1993), p. 14; Mike Mills, "Clinton Technology Policy Aims at Partnership with Industry," *Congressional Quarterly Weekly Report* 51 (February 27, 1993), pp. 453–55; Graeme Browning, "Search for Tomorrow," *National Journal* 25 (March 20, 1993), pp. 674–79.
8. On the awareness of the use of information technology for society's benefit, see especially chapter 4 and also John E. Searles,

"Information Technology and Social Studies," *Social Education* 47 (May 1983), pp. 335–37.

2 Human Knowledge as a Source of Aid and Support

1. On the use of information for the benefit of mankind, see Gunther R. Geiss and Narayan Viswanathan (eds), *The Human Edge: Information Technology and Helping People* (New York: The Haworth Press, 1986); Forester, *Computers in the Human Context*; Frederick Williams and John V. Pavlik (eds), *The People's Right to Know: Media, Democracy and the Information Highway* (Hillsdale, NJ: L. Erlbaum Associates, 1993); V. A. Vinogradov and L. V. Skvorsov, *Information Culture: A Key to Social Development and Improvement of Human Existence* (The Hague: SPB Academic Publishers, 1991).
2. The need for information is particularly emphasized in the health establishment and in the framework of the new "patient education" discipline. An interesting example of the development of information services in the framework of international health services can be found in Great Britain: Michael Brittain, "Information and the Health of the Nation," *Aslib Proceedings* 45(2) (1993), pp. 53–60; W. Abbot (ed.), *Information Technology in Health Care* (Harlow, Essex: Longman, 1992).
3. See R. Gann, "Consumer Health Information," in L. T. Morton and Shane Godbolt (eds), *Information Sources in Medical Sciences*, 4th edn (London: Bowker-Saur, 1992), pp. 545–55.

3 "Mrs Jones" in 1995 and 2025

1. Examples of case studies illustrating the importance of information being used for the public benefit can be found in the proceedings of The Information Technology and Social Work Practice Conference, held in 1984 at Wye Plantation of the Aspen Institute of Humanistic Studies; see Gunther R. Geiss and Narayan Viswanathan, *The Human Edge*. That approach, which views the therapist as an agent helping mankind find the necessary solutions to their problems, emphasizes the importance of self-help; Eliot Freidson, *Profession of Medicine: A Study of the Sociology of Applied Knowledge* (New York: Dodd, Mead, 1970), p. 382: "It is my opinion that the professional's role in a free society should be limited to contributing the technical

information men need to make their own decisions on the basis of their own values."

4 The Heritage of the 20th Century

1. For the history of bibliotherapy and its application in various sciences, see Elenor F. Brown, *Bibliotherapy and its Widening Application* (Metuchen, NJ: Scarecrow Press, 1975); Ruth M. Tews, "Bibliotherapy," in *Encyclopedia of Library and Information Science* 2 (1969), pp. 448–57; Rhea Rubin, *Using Bibliotherapy: A Guide to Theory and Practice* (Phoenix, AZ: Oryx Press, 1978); Rhea Rubin, *Bibliotherapy Source Book* (Phoenix, AZ: Oryx Press, 1978). A list of major studies in bibliotherapy is given in the comprehensive book by Arleen Hynes McCarty and Mary Hynes Berry, *Biblio/Poetry Therapy – The Interactive Process: A Handbook* (Boulder, CO: Westview Press, 1986). For the development of the field of bibliotherapy as part of librarianship, see Alice Gulen Smith, "Whatever Happened to Library Education for Bibliotherapy," *Advances in Library Administration and Organization* 9 (1991), pp. 29–59. For the development of academic research in the field, see Alice Gulen Smith, "The Library Profession in the 21st Century," pp. 37ff. An interesting example of the application of bibliotherapy in the US Veterans Administration libraries can be seen in the activities of the librarian Sadie Peterson Delaney: see Betty K. Gubert, "Sadie Peterson Delaney, Pioneer Bibliotherapist," *American Libraries* 24 (February 1993), pp. 124–30. A comprehensive book on the psychological and educational aspects of bibliotherapy was recently published in Hebrew: Adir Cohen, *Bibliotherapy*, 2 vols (Kiriat Bialik: Ach., 1990). For basic aspects of psychology and bibliotherapy, see the research of two psychologists: Jean Pardeck and John Pardeck, *Young People with Problems* (Westport, CT: Greenwood Press, 1984); and also their book *Bibliotherapy – A Clinical Approach for Helping Children* (Special Aspects of Education 16) (Amsterdam: Gordon & Breach, 1993); Jean M. Clarke and Eileen Bostle, *Reading Therapy* (London: The Library Association, 1988). On the importance of reading to hospital patients, see Mona E. Going and Jean M. Clarke (eds), *Hospital Libraries and Work with the Disabled in the Community*, 3rd edn (London: The Library Association, 1981), pp. 211–36.
2. Caroline Shrodes, "Bibliotherapy, A Theoretical and Clinical

Experimental Study" (Ph.D. dissertation, University of California, 1949).

3. R. L. Barker, *The Social Work Dictionary* (Silver Spring, MD: NASW, 1987).
4. Pardeck and Pardeck, *Bibliotherapy*, p. 7.
5. On doubts as to the effectiveness of bibliotherapy, see Lucy Warner, "The Myth of Bibliotherapy," *School Library Journal* (October 1980), pp. 107–11. For bibliotherapy studies in universities and in the framework of various organizations, see Alice G. Smith, "Whatever Happened to Library Education for Bibliotherapy"; Alice G. Smith, "Will the Real Bibliotherapist Please Stand Up," *Journal of Youth Services in Libraries* 2 (November 1992), pp. 241–49; Hynes, *Biblio/Poetry Therapy*, pp. 247–48. See the Appendix for the Bar-Ilan program.
6. Joseph Gold, *Read for your Life, Literature as a Life Support System* (Markham, Ontario: Fitzhenny & Whiteside, 1990).
7. On the art of story-telling, see Augusta Baker and Ellin Greene, *Storytelling: Art and Technique* (New York: R. R. Bowker, 1977); Caroline Feller Bauer's, *New Handbook for Storytellers* (Chicago: American Library Association, 1993).
8. About the NLP method, see R. Bandler and J. Grinder, *The Structure of Magic* (Palo Alto, CA: Science and Behavior Books, 1975). An interesting application of the NLP theory can be found in Leslie Cameron Bandler, *Solutions: Practical and Effective Antidotes for Sexual and Relationship Problems* (San Rafael, CA: Future Pace, Inc., 1985). On Milton Erickson's methods, see Sidney Rosen (ed.), *My Voice will Go with You, The Teaching Tales of Milton H. Erickson* (New York and London: W.W. Norton, 1982); Jay Haley, *Uncommon Therapy, The Psychiatric Techniques of Milton H. Erickson* (New York and London: W.W. Norton, 1986). For the use of metaphors in the NLP method, see David Gordon, *Therapeutic Metaphors, Helping Others Through the Looking Glass* (Cupertino, CA: META Publications, 1978).
9. Many studies in the field of psychoneuroimmunology have been published over the last few years. Some examples are: Robert Ornstein and David Sobel, *The Healing Brain* (New York: Simon & Schuster, 1987); Norman Cousins, *The Head First, The Biology of Hope* (New York: E. P. Dutton, 1989). M. F. La Via and E. A. Workman, "Psychoneuroimmunology: Yesterday, Today and Tomorrow," *Acta Neurologica* 13 (August 1991),

pp. 335–42; Lawrence T. Vollhardt, "Psychoneuroimmunology: A Literature Review," *American Journal of Orthopsychiatry* 61 (January 1991), pp. 35–47.

10. See A. M. Rees, *Managing Consumer Health Information Services* (Phoenix, AZ: Oryx Press, 1991), p. 18. On the effectiveness and usefulness of self-help books and booklets, see A. Ellis, "The Advantages and Disadvantages of Self-Help Therapy Material," *Professional Psychology – Research and Practice* 24 (August 1993), pp. 335–39; J. A. Marx *et al.*, "Use of Self-Help Books in Psychotherapy," *Professional Psychology – Research and Practice* 23 (August 1992), pp. 300–5; A. J. Blair *et al.*, "Response to Leaflets about Eating and Shape by Women Concerned about their Weight," *Behavioral Psychotherapy* 20 (1992), pp. 279–86; Stephen Hunt, "The Clinical Use of Self Help Manuals," in J. M. Clarke and E. Bostle (eds), *Reading Therapy* (London: The Library Association, 1988), pp. 82–105. The phenomenon of self-help books is related to the phenomenon of the development of the field of patient education: see D. Tolsma, "Patient Education Objectives in Healthy People 2000 – Policy and Research Issues," *Patient Education and Counseling* 22 (November 1993), pp. 7–14.
11. See Gann, "Consumer Health Information," pp. 553–55.
12. Alfred J. Kahn *et al.*, *Neighborhood Information Centers: A Study and Some Proposals* (New York: Columbia University of Social Work, 1966).
13. Thomas Childers, *Information and Referral: Public Libraries* (Norwood, NJ: Ablex Publishing, 1983).
14. Sally Knight, "Health Information in Hospitals and in Community," in Jean M. Clarke and Mona E. Going (eds), *Hospital Libraries and Community Care*, 4th edn (London: The Library Association, 1990), pp. 144–55.
15. See Salvinija G. Kernaghn and Barbara E. Giloth, *Consumer Health Information Managing Hospital-based Centers* (Chicago: American Hospital Association, 1991), p. 1. On the patients' need for information and the activities set up to assist them, see Rebecca R. Martin, "Library and Health Information Services for Patients," in Jana Bradely *et al.* (eds), *Hospital Library Management* (Chicago: Medical Library Association, 1983), pp. 353–65; Ellen Gartenfeld, "Community Access to Health Information Services Hospital Library Management," in Jana Bradely *et al.* (eds), *Hospital Library Management* (Chicago: Medical Library

Association, 1983), pp. 367–79; Judith Callaghan, "Setting Up a Health Information Service in a Hospital Library: Some Practical Considerations," in J. M. Clarke and M. E. Going (eds), *Hospital Libraries and Community Care*, 4th edn (London: The Library Association, 1990), pp. 156–60. About the situation in Israel, see S. Baruchson-Arbib, "The Awareness of 'Aid through the Use of Books and Information' in Medical and Social Institutions in Israel," Bücher als Magische Medizin. *Zum Verständnis des Therapeutischen Potentials bei Kindern und Jugendlichen* (in press – German).

16. Neel Parikh and Marcia Schneider, "Book Buddies, Bringing Stories to Hospitalized Children," *School Library Journal* 35 (December 1988), pp. 35–39; Marcia Schneider, *Book Buddies Volunteers Bring Stories to San Francisco Hospitalized Children – A Manual* (San Francisco: San Francisco Library, 1987).
17. The information on the activities of the German Project was relayed to me by Dr Edith Mundt and Dr Carol Adeney during my visits to Germany in 1991 and 1992. For comprehensive academic research on this project, see Carol Adeney, *Bibliotherapie bei Kleinkindern im Krankenhaus* (*Europäische Hochschulschriften*, Vol. 418) (Frankfurt am Main: Peter Lang, 1990).
18. Joseph J. Lazzaro, *Adaptive Technologies for Learning Work Environments* (Chicago and London: American Library Association, 1993); Jean M. Clarke, "Reading Aids," in J. M. Clarke and M. E. Going (eds), *Hospital Libraries and Community Care*, 4th edn (London: The Library Association, 1990), pp. 176–93; see also Bill Anderson, "Deaf and Hearing Impaired People," in Clarke and Going, *Hospital Libraries and Community Care*, pp. 241–56; David A. Matthews, "Visually Impaired and Disabled People," in Clarke and Going, *Hospital Libraries and Community Care*, pp. 224–40; Julie Ryder, "Library Services to Elderly People and People with Disabilities," in Clarke and Going, *Hospital Libraries and Community Care*, pp. 206–23; Margaret R. Marshall, "Special Reading Material for Handicapped Children," in J. M. Clarke and E. Bostle (eds), *Reading Therapy* (London: The Library Association, 1988), pp. 106–26. A new journal has recently appeared which could greatly facilitate the location of assistance available for the disabled: see *Information Technology and Disabilities*, ed. Tom McNulty, Vol. 1, No. 1 (January 1994). On the use of modern technologies by hospital personnel in

order to expedite information receipt and improve the quality of patient care, see Patrick F. Abrami and Joyce E. Johnson, *Bringing Computers to the Hospital Bedside – An Emerging Technology* (New York: Springer Publishing, 1990).

5 A New Scientific Discipline

1. This information can be found in national bibliographies, such as *Books in Print*, and in library catalogs, such as that of The Library of Congress. Subject catalogs can be found in data bases for health and medical problems. A data base which deserves special mention is the "Burrels Broadcast Database," which contains full text transcripts of national radio and television programs.
2. Bibliographies recommending books according to subject analysis can be found in the following studies: Hynes, *Biblio/Poetry Therapy*, pp. 109–13; Pardeck and Pardeck, *Bibliotherapy*; R. B. Tabor and J. Stephenson, *Reflection: A Subject Guide to Fiction and Biography on Illness and Disability*, 3rd edn (Southampton: Wessex Regional Library Information Service, 1989); Paula Kay Montgomery, *Approaches to Literature through Subject* (The Oryx Reading Motivation Series, 3) (Phoenix, AZ: Oryx Press, 1993).
3. Information concerning ongoing projects can be found by setting up electronic discussion groups.
4. Modern data bases are the basic tool for finding theoretical statistics, and especially the social science citation index. But it should not be forgotten that most of the electronic data bases only contain studies from 1980 onwards. There were many important studies with significant results prior to the 1980s. These studies can be looked up using the conventional reference tools: psychological abstracts, sociological abstracts, Library and Information Science abstracts, and others.
5. For Bar-Ilan University's curriculum, see Appendix.
6. For the development of the study of Librarianship and Information Science, see Antony Debons, "Education in Library and Information Science," *Encyclopedia of Library and Information Science* 7 (1972), pp. 414–74; Abdelhamid Miski, "Education for Information Science," *Encyclopedia of Library and Information Science* 41 (1986), pp. 47–65; Susan K. Martin, "Information Technology and Libraries; Toward the Year 2000," *College*

and Research Libraries 50 (July 1989), pp. 397–405; April Bohannan, "Library Education: Struggling to Meet the Needs of the Profession," *Journal of Academic Librarianship* 17 (September 1991), pp. 216–19; Metro Voloshin, "The Information Revolution and the Library Community, The Good and Bad," *West Virginia Libraries* 41 (Summer 1988), pp. 10–13; Bruce Park, "Libraries without Walls; or, Librarians without a Profession," *American Libraries* 23 (October 1982), pp. 746–47; Mary L. Smalls, "The Library Profession in the 21st Century: Transformation for Survival," paper presented at the Annual Meeting of Georgia Library Association, Augusta, GA: October 25, 1985; Michael Garman, "The Academic Library in the Year 2001: Dream or Nightmare or Something in Between?" *The Journal of Academic Librarianship* 17 (1991), pp. 4–9. See also C. D. Hurt, "Future of Library Science in Higher Education," *Advances in Librarianship* 16 (1992), pp. 153–81; Margaret F. Stieg, *Change and Challenge in Library and Information Science Education* (Chicago: American Library Association, 1992).

6 The Future *SI Scientist*

1. The Bar-Ilan curriculum for Information and Society can be used as an initial model for training Information scientists. Basic concepts on the educational background of Social Information scientists can also be found in studies dealing with the training of bibliotherapists, for example: Arleen McCarty Hynes, "Certification in the St. Elizabeth's Hospital Bibliotherapy Training Program," in Rhea J. Rubin, *Using Bibliotherapy: A Guide to Theory and Practice* (Phoenix, AZ: Oryx Press, 1978), pp. 201–12; Morris R. Morrison, "Standards for Certification of Poetry Therapists and Related Matters: A Proposal," in Rhea J. Rubin, *Using Bibliotherapy*, pp. 213–16; Margaret M. Kinney, "The Bibliotherapy Program: Requirements for Training," *Library Trends* 11 (October 1962), pp. 127–37.
2. On the bibliotherapeutic activities at St Elizabeth's Hospital, see Arleen McCarty Hynes, "Bibliotherapy in the Circulating Library at St. Elizabeth's Hospital," in Rhea J. Rubin (ed.), *Bibliotherapy Source Book* (Phoenix, AZ: Oryx Press, 1978), pp. 300–4.
3. On the need for Information in aid organizations, see Shifra Baruchson-Arbib, "Information and Supportive Literature in Aid Organizations" (in press). In a survey conducted among

aid organizations in Israel in 1994, it was found that 61.2 percent have no libraries and that 100 percent are in favor of the development of information and library services.

4. On the cost of information, see Kenneth John Bierman, "Cost of Electronic Information," *Encyclopedia of Library and Information Science* 54 (1994), pp. 122–43. On the threat to privacy in the Information Age, see Large, *The Micro Revolution*, pp. 163–73.

7 Establishing the New Discipline

1. On preventive medicine and its promotion through the media, see D. Tolsma, "Patient Education"; Edward A. Brawley, *Mass Media and Human Services: Getting the Message Across* (Beverly Hills: Sage Publications, 1983).
2. See Michael L. Baizerman, "Hotline Research: Critique, Response and Rejoinder," *Professional Psychology* 7 (May 1976), pp. 236–39; Gail A. Bleach, "An Evolution of Hotline Services, Process and Outcome," Ph.D. dissertation, University of Maryland, 1975; Alan Rosenbaum and James P. Calhoun, "The Use of the Telephone Hotline in Crisis Intervention: A Review," *Journal of Community Psychology* 5 (October 1977), pp. 325–39; U. Delworth *et al.*, *Crisis Center – Hotline: A Guidebook to Beginning and Operating* (Springfield: Charles C. Thomas, 1972).
3. See Rubin, *Using Bibliotherapy*, p. 8. For Nicholas Rubakin's theory on bibliopsychology, see Sylva Simsova, "Nicholas Rubakin and Bibliopsychology," in Rhea J. Rubin (ed.), *Bibliotherapy Source Book*, pp. 354–65.
4. For example, selected references for locating bibliotherapeutic material can be found in Hynes, *Biblio/Poetry Therapy*, pp. 110–13.
5. While it is possible to use the basic classification methods such as Dewey and the Library of Congress Subject Heading, these methods do not emphasize the therapeutic elements. For simple classification according to general subjects, see chapter 5, note 3.
6. An example of an original classification is the classification method used by the National Committee for Hospital Libraries created by the Belgian Red Cross, see *Librarianship and Therapy: Hospital and Handicapped Readers Group Conference*, 1967

(London: The Library Association, 1968). The questionnaire mentioned above was based on a model suggested by Cohen (*Bibliotherapy*, pp. 151ff), but the chosen model does not include the hypertext approach.

7. On the importance of using biographies in the bibliotherapeutic process, see Cohen, *Bibliotherapy*, pp. 133–37.
8. See Carl Simonton *et al.*, *Getting Well Again* (New York: Bantam, 1980); Bernie S. Siegel, *Love, Medicine and Miracles* (New York: Harper and Row, 1986); Blair Justice, *Think yourself Healthy: How Thoughts, Moods and Beliefs can Affect your Health* (Wellingborough, Northamptonshire: Thorsons Publishers, 1989); James V. Van Camp, "Modification of Adult Aggressive Behavior by Using Modeling Films," Ph.D. dissertation, Pasadena, CA: Fuller Theological Seminary Graduate School of Psychology, 1972.
9. On the popularity of computer games and their social role: Eric A. Agli and Lawrence S. Meyers, "The Role of Video Game Playing in Adolescent Life, Is There a Reason to be Concerned?" *Bulletin of the Psychonomic Society* 22 (1984), pp. 309–12; Nicola S. Schutte, "Effects of Playing Video Games on Children's Aggressive and Other Behaviours," *Journal ofApplied Social Psychology* 18 (April 1988), pp. 454–60.
10. On the effectiveness of using hypnosis and guided imagery, see Ms Torem, "The Use of Hypnosis with Eating Disorders," *Psychiatric Medicine* 10 (1992), pp. 105–18; R. Zachariae *et al.*, "Effect of Psychological Intervention in the Form of Relaxation and Guided Imagery on Cellular Immune Function in Normal Healthy Subjects: An Overview," *Psychoter. Psychosom.* 54 (1990), pp. 32–39.
11. See G. Makari and T. Shapiro, "On Psychoanalytic Listening: Language and Unconscious Communication," *Journal of American Psychoanalysis Association* 41 (1993), pp. 991–1020; N. Dixon and C. Henley, "Unconscious Perception, Possible Implications of Data from Academic Research for Clinical Practice," *Journal of Nervous and Mental Disease* 179 (May 1991), pp. 243–52; Jean Marc Nores *et al.*, "Some Problems Involving Perception under Anaesthesia: The Contribution of Hypnosis to the Understanding of the Ego," *Australian Journal of Clinical and Experimental Hypnosis* 17 (November 1989), pp. 163–65; Edwin K. Yager, "Subliminal Therapy Utilizing the Unconscious Mind," *Medicine Hypnoanalysis Journal* 2 (December 1987),

pp. 138–47; Hans Carl Leuner, "Guided Effective Imagery: An Account of its Development," *Journal of Mental Imagery* 1 (Spring 1977), pp. 73–91. About Émile Coué, see C. H. Brooks, *The Practice of Autosuggestion by the Method of Émile Coué* (rev. edn) (New York: Dodd, Mead, 1922).

12. See Brawley, *Mass Media and Human Services*; Liz Hodgkinson, *Smile Therapy: How Smiling and Laughter can Change your Life* (London: MacDonald, 1987).
13. Shifra Baruchson-Arbib, "Self-help Section in the Modern Public Library" (in press).
14. See Gold, *Read for your Life*, pp. 360–67.
15. On the economic value of the information revolution, see Edward J. Malecki, "High Tech and Economic Development: Hope or Hype?" in Tom Forester (ed.), *Computers in the Human Context*, pp. 462–67.
16. On the role of the library and reading in improving the life of the elderly, see Martin Skelton Robinson, "Ageing and the Interests of the Elderly, With Special Reference to Reading," in J. M. Clarke and E. Bostle (eds), *Reading Therapy*, pp. 163–79; on the importance of self-confidence and motivation in the life of the elderly in modern society, see Paul Thompson, "I Don't Feel Old: The Significance of the Search for Meaning in Later Life," *International Journal of Geriatric Psychiatry* 8 (August 1993), pp. 685–92; Michael J. Siebers *et al.*, *Coping with Loss of Independence* (San Diego, CA: Singular Publishing Group, 1993; Eleanor L. Swartz, "The Older Adult: Creative Use of Leisure Time," *Journal of Geriatric Psychiatry* 11 (1978), pp. 85–87; Esther E. Twente, *Never Too Old: The Aged in Community Life* (San Francisco, CA: Jossey Bass, 1970); Robert M. Kaplan *et al.*, "Patient Information Processing and the Decision to Accept Treatment," *Journal of Social Behavior and Personality* (January 1985), pp. 113–20.
17. See Toffler, *War and Anti-war*, chaps 16, 18.

8 Academic Research, Basic Theories and Questions

1. On the theory of "Livre et Société," see R. Birn, "Livre et Société after Ten Years: Formation of a Discipline," *Studies on Voltaire and the Eighteenth Century* 151 (1976), pp. 287–312; Shifra Baruchson-Arbib, "Nuova bibliologia e storia del libro ebraico," *Annuario di studi ebraici* 10 (1980–84), pp. 17–28.

The book by L. Febvre and H. J. Martin was translated into English by D. Gerard: *The Coming of the Book – The Impact of Printing 1450–1800* (London: NLB, 1976). For an example of the application of the theory of Livre et Société, see Shifra Baruchson-Arbib, *Books and Readers – The Reading Interests of the Italian Jews at the Close of the Renaissance* (Ramat Gan: Bar-Ilan University Press, 1993) (Hebrew).

2. For examples of research on information needs and factors influencing the interest in and use of information, see M. C. Shapiro and J. M. Najman, "Socio-economic Status Differences in Patients' Desire for Capacity to Obtain Information in Clinical Encounter," *Australian Journal of Social Issues* 22 (May 1987), pp. 465–71; Mary F. Backlin Mohammed, "Patients' Understanding of Written Health Information," *Nursing Research* 13 (Spring 1964), pp. 100–8.
3. The way information should be conveyed to the consumer or patient can be learned from studies in medicine and psychology, for example: Fredric M. Wolf *et al.*, "A Controlled Experiment in Teaching Students to Respond to Patients' Emotional Concerns," *Journal of Medical Education* 62 (January 1987), pp. 25–34; H. Spiro, "What is Empathy and can it be Taught," *Annals of Internal Medicine* 116 (May 1992), pp. 843–46.
4. For examples of problems emerging in the information-giving process, see Geiss and Viswanathan, *The Human Edge*; Large, *The Micro Revolution*.
5. See David Nicholas and Maureen Ritchie, *Literature and Bibliometrics* (London: Clive Bingley, 1978); Christine L. Borgman (ed.), *Title Scholarly Communication and Bibliometrics* (Newbury Park: Sage, 1990).

Bibliography

Abbot W. (ed.), *Information Technology in Health Care*, Harlow, Essex: Longman, 1992.

Abrami, Patrick F. and Johnson, Joyce E., *Bringing Computers to the Hospital Bedside – An Emerging Technology*, New York: Springer Publishing Company, 1990.

Adeney, Carol, *Bibliotherapie bei Kleinkindern in Krankenhaus,* (*Europäische Hochschulschriften*, Vol. 418), Frankfurt am Main: Peter Lang, 1990.

Anderson, Bill, "Deaf and Hearing Impaired People," in: J. M. Clarke and M. E. Going (eds), *Hospital Libraries and Community Care*, 4th edn, London: The Library Association, 1990, pp. 241–56.

Baizerman, Michael L., "Hotline Research: Critique, Response and Rejoinder," *Professional Psychology* 7 (May 1976), pp. 236–39.

Baker, Augusta and Greene, Ellin, *Storytelling: Art and Technique*, New York: R. R. Bowker, 1977.

Bandler, R. and Grinder, J., *The Structure of Magic*, Palo Alto, CA: Science and Behavior Books, 1975.

Bankes, Steve *et al.*, "Harnessing the Information Technologies," *Information Society* 8 (January 1992), pp. 1–59.

Barker, R. L., *The Social Work Dictionary*, Silver Spring, MD: NASW, 1987.

Baruchson-Arbib, Shifra, "The Awareness of 'Aid through the use of Books and Information' in Medical and Social Institutions in Israel," Bücher als Magische Medizin. *Zum Verständnis des Therapeutischen Potentials bei Kindern und Jugendlichen* (in press – German).

——, *Books and Readers – The Reading Interests of the Italian Jews at the Close of the Renaissance*, Ramat Gan: Bar-Ilan University

Press, 1993 (Hebrew).

——, "Information and Supportive Literature in Aid Organizations" (in press).

——, "Nuova bibliologia e storia del libro ebraico," *Annuario di studi ebraici* 10 (1980–84), pp. 17–28.

——, "Self-Help Section in the Modern Public Library" (in press).

Bauer's Caroline Feller, *New Handbook for Storytellers*, Chicago: American Library Association, 1993.

Bequai, August, *Technocrimes*, Lexington, MA: Lexington Books, 1987.

Bierman, Kenneth John, "Cost of Electronic Information," *Encyclopedia of Library and Information Science* 54 (1994), pp. 122–43.

Birn, R., "Livre et Société After Ten Years: Formation of a Discipline," *Studies on Voltaire and the Eighteenth Century* 151 (1976), pp. 287–312.

Blair, A. J. *et al.*, "Response to Leaflets about Eating and Shape by Women Concerned about their Weight," *Behavioral Psychotherapy* 20 (1992), pp. 279–86.

Bleach, Gail A., "An Evaluation of Hotline Services, Process and Outcome," Ph.D. dissertation, University of Maryland, 1975.

Bohannan, April, "Library Education: Struggling to Meet the Needs of the Profession," *Journal of Academic Librarianship* 17 (September 1991), pp. 216–19.

Borgman, Christine L. (ed.), *Title Scholarly Communication and Bibliometrics*, Newbury Park: Sage, 1990.

Brawley, Edward A., *Mass Media and Human Services: Getting the Message Across*, Beverly Hills: Sage Publications, 1983.

Brittain, Michael, "*Information and the Health of the Nation*," Aslib Proceedings 45(2) (1993), pp. 53–60.

Brod, C., *Technostress: The Human Cost of the Computer Revolution*, Reading, MA: Addison-Wesley, 1984.

Brooks, C. H., *The Practice of Autosuggestion by the Method of Émile Coué* (rev. edn), New York: Dodd, Mead, 1922.

Brown, Elenor F., *Bibliotherapy and its Widening Application*, Metuchen, NJ: Scarecrow Press, 1975.

Browning, Graeme, "Search for Tomorrow," *National Journal* 25 (March 20, 1993), pp. 674–79.

Callaghan, Judith, "Setting up a Health Information Service in a Hospital Library: Some Practical Considerations," in J. M. Clarke and M. E. Going (eds), *Hospital Libraries and Community Care*, 4th edn, London: The Library Association, 1990, pp. 156–60.

Cameron Bandler, Leslie, *Solutions, Practical and Effective Antidotes for Sexual and Relationship Problems*, San Rafael, CA: Future Pace, Inc., 1985.

Childers, Thomas, *Information and Referral: Public Libraries*, Norwood, NJ: Ablex Publishing Co., 1983.

Cohen, Adir, *Bibliotherapy*, 2 vols, Kiriat Bialik: Ach, 1990 (Hebrew).

Clarke, Jean M., "Reading Aids," in J. M. Clarke and M. E. Going (eds), *Hospital Libraries and Community Care*, 4th edn, London: The Library Association, 1990, pp. 176–93.

Clarke, Jean M. and Bostle, Eileen, *Reading Therapy*, London: The Library Association, 1988.

Cooper, Marc, "New Horizons: Clinton's Technology Policy and the Project Information Superhighway," *Bulletin of the Israel Society of Special Libraries and Information Centers* 19 (May 1993), pp. 43–44.

Cousins, Norman, *The Head First: The Biology of Hope*, New York: E. P. Dutton, 1989.

Davidson, Robert S. and Wally, Page B., "Computer Fear and Addiction: Analysis, Prevention and Possible Modification," *Journal of Organizational Behaviour Management* 6 (1984), pp. 37–51.

Debons, Anthony, "Education in Library and Information Science," *Encyclopedia of Library and Information Science* 7 (1972), pp. 414–74.

Delworth, U. *et al.*, *Crisis Center – Hotline: A Guidebook to Beginning and Operating*, Springfield: Charles C. Thomas, 1972.

Dixon, N. and Henley, C., "Unconscious Perception. Possible Implications of Data from Academic Research for Clinical Practice," *Journal of Nervous and Mental Disease* 179 (May 1991), pp. 243–52.

Egli, Eric A. and Meyers, Lawrence S., "The Role of Video Game Playing in Adolescent Life, Is There a Reason to be Concerned?" *Bulletin of the Psychonomic Society* 22 (1984), pp. 309–12.

Eisenstein, Elizabeth L., *The Printing Press as an Agent of Change*, Cambridge: Cambridge University Press, 1979.

Ellis, A., "The Advantages and Disadvantages of Self-Help Therapy Material," *Professional Psychology – Research and Practice* 24 (August 1993), pp. 335–39.

Febvre, Lucien and Martin, Henri Jean, *The Coming of the Book: The Impact of Printing, 1450–1800*, London: NLB, 1976.

Forester, Tom (ed.), *Computers in the Human Context*, Oxford: Basil Blackwell, 1989.

Freidson, Eliot, *Profession of Medicine: A Study of the Sociology of Applied Knowledge*, New York: Dodd, Mead, 1970.

Gann, R., "Consumer Health Information," in L. T. Morton and Shane Godbolt (eds), *Information Sources in Medical Sciences*, 4th edn, London: Bowker-Sauer, 1992, pp. 545–55.

Garman, Michael, "The Academic Library in the Year 2001: Dream or Nightmare or Something in Between?" *The Journal of Academic Librarianship* 17 (1991), pp. 4–9.

Gartenfeld, Ellen, "Community Access to Health Information Services," in J. Bradely *et al.* (eds), *Hospital Library Management*, Chicago: Medical Library Association, 1985, pp. 367–79.

Geiss, Gunther, R. and Viswanathan, Narayan (eds), *The Human Edge: Information Technology and Helping People*, New York: The Haworth Press, 1986.

Going, Mona E. and Clarke, Jean M. (eds), *Hospital Libraries and Work with the Disabled in the Community*, 3rd edn, London: The Library Association, 1981.

Gold, Joseph, *Read for your Life, Literature as a Life Support System*, Markham, Ontario: Fitzhenry & Whiteside, 1990.

Gordon, David, *Therapeutic Metaphors, Helping Others Through the Looking Glass*, Cupertino, CA: META Publications, 1978.

Gore, Al, "Infrastructure for the Global Village," *Scientific American* 265 (September 1991), pp. 150–53.

Gubert, Betty K., "Sadie Peterson Delaney: Pioneer Bibliotherapist," *American Libraries* 24 (February 1993), pp. 124–30.

Haley, Jay, *Uncommon Therapy of Psychiatric Techniques of Milton H. Erickson*, New York and London: W.W. Norton, 1986.

Hodgkinson, Liz, *Smile Therapy: How Smiling and Laughter can Change your Life*, London: Macdonald, 1987.

Howitt, D. and Cumberbatch, G., *Mass Media, Violence and Society*, London: Elek Science, 1975.

Hunt, Stephen, "The Clinical Use of Self Help Manuals," in J. M. Clarke and E. Bostle (eds), *Reading Therapy*, London: The Library Association, 1988, pp. 82–105.

Hurt, C. D., "Future of Library Science in Higher Education," *Advances in Librarianship* 16 (1992), pp. 153–81.

Hynes Arleen, McCarty, "Bibliotherapy in the Circulating Library at St. Elizabeth's Hospital," in Rhea J. Rubin, *Bibliotherapy Source Book*, Phoenix, AZ: Oryx Press, 1978, pp. 300–4.

——, "Certification in the St. Elizabeth's Hospital Bibliotherapy Training Program," in Rhea J. Rubin, *Using Bibliotherapy: A*

Guide to Theory and Practice, Phoenix, AZ: Oryx Press, 1978, pp. 201–12.

Hynes Arleen, McCarty and Hynes, Mary Berry, *Biblio/Poetry Therapy – The Interactive Process: A Handbook*, Boulder, CO: Westview Press, 1986.

Justice, Blair, *Think yourself Healthy: How Beliefs, Moods and Thoughts can Affect your Health*, Wellingborough, Northamptonshire: Thorsons, 1989.

Kahn, Alfred J. *et al.*, *Neighborhood Information Centers: A Study and Some Proposals*, New York: Columbia University of Social Work, 1966.

Kaplan, Robert M. *et al.*, "Patient Information Processing and the Decision to Accept Treatment," *Journal of Social Behavior and Personality* 1 (January 1985), pp. 113–20.

Kernaghn, Salvinija and Giloth, Barbara E., *Consumer Health Information Managing Hospital-based Centers*, Chicago: American Hospital Association, 1991.

Kinney, Margaret M., "The Bibliotherapy Program: Requirements for Training," *Library Trends* 11 (October 1962), pp. 127–37.

Knight, Sally, "Health Information in Hospitals and in Community," in Jean M. Clarke and Mona E. Going (eds), *Hospital Libraries and Community Care*, 4th edn, London: The Library Association, 1990, pp. 144–55.

La Via, M. F. and Workman, E. A., "Psychoneuroimmunology: Yesterday, Today and Tomorrow," *Acta Neurologica* 13 (August 1991), pp. 335–42.

Lancaster, F. W., *Toward Paperless Information Systems*, New York: Academic Press, 1978.

Lankes, R. D., "National Net 1993 Conference Explores Information Superhighway under Clinton Administration," *Library Hi Tech News* 104 (July–August 1993), p. 14.

Lanquey, Tracy and Ryer, Jeanne C., *The Internet Companion – A Beginner's Guide to Global Networking*, Reading, MA: Addison Wesley, 1993.

Large, Peter, *The Micro Revolution Revisited*, London: Frances Pinter, 1984.

Laurie, P., *The Micro Revolution: A Change for the Better or for the Worse?* New York: Futura Publications, 1980.

Lazzaro, Joseph J., *Adaptive Technologies for Learning Work Environments*, Chicago and London: American Library Association, 1993.

Lee, James K., "Toward the Information Superhighway," *Telecommunication Policy* 17 (November 1993), pp. 631–35.

Leuner, Hans Carl, "Guided Effective Imagery: An Account of its Development," *Journal of Mental Imagery* 1 (Spring 1977), pp. 73–91.

Librarianship and Therapy: Hospital and Handicapped Readers Group Conference (1967), London: The Library Association, 1968.

Makari, G. and Shapiro, T., "On Psychoanalytic Listening: Language and Unconscious Communication," *Journal of American Psychoanalysis Association* 41 (1993), pp. 991–1020.

Malecki, Edward J., "High Tech and Economic Development: Hope or Hype?" in Tom Forester (ed.), *Computers in the Human Context*, Oxford: Basil Blackwell, 1989, pp. 462–67.

Marshall, Margaret R., "Special Reading Material for Handicapped Children," in J. M. Clarke and E. Bostle (eds), *Reading Therapy*, London: The Library Association, 1988, pp. 106–26.

Martin, Rebecca R., "Library and Health Information Services for Patients," in Jana Bradely *et al.* (eds), *Hospital Library Management*, Chicago: Medical Library Association, 1983, pp. 353–65.

Martin, Susan K., "Information Technology and Libraries: Toward the Year 2000," *College and Research Libraries* 50 (July 1989), pp. 397–405.

Marx, Gary A. and Sherizen, Sanford, "Monitoring on the Job," in Tom Forester (ed.), *Computers in the Human Context*, Oxford: Basil Blackwell, 1989, pp. 397–406.

Marx, J. A. *et al.*, "Use of Self-Help Books in Psychotherapy," *Professional Psychology – Research and Practice* 23 (August 1992), pp. 300–5.

Matthews, David A., "Visually Impaired and Disabled People," in J. M. Clarke and M. E. Going (eds), *Hospital Libraries and Community Care*, 4th edn, London: The Library Association, 1990, pp. 224–40.

McGary, Kevin, *The Changing Context of Information, An Introductory Analysis*, 2nd edn, London: Library Association Publishing, 1993.

Meir, Alexandra, "The Gutenberg Project," *Bulletin of the Israel Society of Special Libraries and Information Centers* 19 (May 1993), pp. 33–35 (Hebrew).

Mills, Mike, "Clinton Technology Policy Aims at Partnership with Industry," *Congressional Quarterly Weekly Report* 51 (February

27, 1993), pp. 453–55.

Miski, Abdelhamid, "Education for Information Science," *Encyclopedia of Library and Information Science* 41 (1986), pp. 47–65.

Mohammed, Mary F. Backlin, "Patients' Understanding of Written Health Information," *Nursing Research* 13 (Spring 1964), pp. 100–8.

Montgomery, Paula Kay, *Approaches to Literature through Subject* (The Oryx Reading Motivation Series, 3) Phoenix, AZ: Oryx Press, 1993.

Morrison, Morris R., "Standards for Certification of Poetry Therapists and Related Matters: A Proposal," in Rhea J. Rubin, *Using Bibliotherapy: A Guide to Theory and Practice*, Phoenix, AZ: Oryx Press, 1978, pp. 213–16.

Nelson, Theodor H., "Electronic Publishing and Electronic Literature," in Edward C. Deland, *Information Technology in Health Science Education*, New York and London: Plenum Press, 1978, pp. 211–16.

New Horizons, "Clinton's Technology Policy and the Prospect for Information Superhighway," *Bulletin of the Israel Society of Special Libraries and Information Centers* 19 (May 1993), pp. 43–44.

Nicholas, David and Ritchie, Maureen, *Literature and Bibliometrics*, London: Clive Bingley, 1978.

Nores, Jean Marc *et al.*, "Some Problems Involving Perceptions under Anaesthesia; The Contribution of Hypnosis to the Understanding of the Ego," *Australian Journal of Clinical and Experimental Hypnosis* 17 (November 1989), pp. 163–65.

Ornstein, Robert and Sobel, David, *The Healing Brain*, New York: Simon & Schuster, 1987.

Pardeck, Jean A. and Pardeck, John T., *Bibliotherapy – A Clinical Approach for Helping Children* (Special Aspects of Education: 16), Amsterdam: Gordon & Breach, 1993.

——, *Young People with Problems*, Westport, CT: Greenwood Press, 1984.

Parikh, Neel and Schneider, Marcia, "Book Buddies, Bringing Stories to Hospitalized Children," *School Library Journal* 35 (December 1988), pp. 35–39.

Park, Bruce, "Libraries without Walls; Or, Librarians without a Profession," *American Libraries* 23 (October 1982), pp. 746–47.

Rees, A. M., *Managing Consumer Health Information Services*, Phoenix, AZ: Oryx Press, 1991.

Robinson, Martin Skelton, "Ageing and the Interest of the Elderly with Special References to Reading," in J. M. Clarke and E. Bostle (eds), *Reading Therapy*, London: The Library Association, 1988, pp. 163–79.

Rosen, Sidney (ed.), *My Voice will Go with You, The Teaching Tales of Milton H. Erickson*, New York and London: W.W. Norton, 1982.

Rosenbaum, Alan and Calhoun, James F., "The Use of the Telephone Hotline in Crisis Intervention: A Review," *Journal of Community Psychology* 5 (October 1977), pp. 325–39.

Rubin, Rhea, *Bibliotherapy Source Book*, Phoenix, AZ: Oryx Press, 1978.

——, *Using Bibliotherapy: A Guide to Theory and Practice*, Phoenix, AZ: Oryx Press, 1978.

Ryder, Julie, "Library Services to Elderly People and People with Disabilities," in J. M. Clarke and M. E. Going (eds), *Hospital Libraries and Community Care*, 4th edn, London: The Library Association, 1990, pp. 206–23.

Schneider, Marcia, *Book Buddies Volunteers Bring Stories to San Francisco Hospitalized Children*, San Francisco: San Francisco Library, 1987.

Schutte, Nicola S., "Effects of Playing Video Games on Children's Aggressive and other Behaviours," *Journal of Applied Social Psychology* 18 (April 1988), pp. 454–60.

Searles, John E., "Information Technology and Social Studies," *Social Education* 47 (May 1983), pp. 335–37.

Shapiro, M. C. and Najman, J. M., "Socio-economic Status Differences in Patients' Desire for Capacity to Obtain Information in Clinical Encounter," *Australian Journal of Social Issues* 22 (May 1987), pp. 465–71.

Shotton, Margaret A., *Computer Addiction? A Study of Computer Dependency*, London: Taylor & Francis, 1989.

——, "The Cost and Benefit of Computer Addiction," *Behaviour and Information Technology* 10 (1991), pp. 219–30.

Shrodes, Caroline, "Bibliotherapy, A Theoretical and Clinical Experimental Study", Ph.D. dissertation, University of California, 1949.

Siebers, Michael J. *et al.*, *Coping with Loss of Independence*, San Diego, CA: Singular Publishing Group, 1993.

Siegel, Bernie S., *Love, Medicine and Miracles*, New York: Harper & Row, 1986.

Simonton, Carl *et al.*, *Getting Well Again*, New York: Bantam, 1980.

Simsova, Sylva, "Nicholas Rubakin and Bibliopsychology," in Rhea J. Rubin (ed.), *Bibliotherapy Source Book*, Phoenix, AZ: Oryx Press, 1978, pp. 354–65.

Smalls, Mary L., "The Library Profession in the 21st Century: Transformation for Survival." Paper presented at the Annual Meeting of Georgia Library Association, Augusta, GA, October 25, 1985.

Smith, Alice Gulen, "Whatever Happened to Library Education for Bibliotherapy?" *Advances in Library Administration and Organization* 9 (1991), pp. 29–59.

——, "Will the Real Bibliotherapist Please Stand Up?" *Journal of Youth Services in Libraries* 2 (November 1989), pp. 241–49.

Spiro, H., "What is Empathy and can it be Taught?" *Annals of Internal Medicine* 116 (May 1992), pp. 843–46.

Stieg, Margaret F., *Change and Challenge in Library and Information Science Education*, Chicago: American Library Association, 1992.

Swartz, Eleanor L., "The Older Adult: Creative use of Leisure Time," *Journal of Geriatric Psychiatry* 11 (1978), pp. 85–87.

Tabor, R. B. and Stephenson, J., *Reflections: A Subject Guide to Fiction and Biography on Illness and Disability*, 3rd edn, Southampton: Wessex Regional Library Information Service, 1989.

Tews, Ruth M., "Bibliotherapy," in *Encyclopedia of Library and Information Science* 2 (1969), pp. 448–57.

Thompson, Paul, "'I Don't Feel Old': The Significance of the Search for Meaning in Later Life," *International Journal of Geriatric Psychiatry* 8 (August 1993), pp. 685–92.

Toffler, Alvin, *Powershift: Knowledge, Wealth and Violence at the Edge of the 21st Century*, New York: Bantam Books, 1990.

Toffler, Alvin and Heidi, *War and Anti-War; Survival at the Dawn of the 21st Century*, Boston: Little Brown, 1993.

Tolsma, D., "Patient Education Objectives in Healthy People 2000 – Policy and Research Issues," *Patient Education and Counseling* 22 (November 1993), pp. 7–14.

Torem, Ms., "The Use of Hypnosis with Eating Disorders," *Psychiatric Medicine* 10 (1992), pp. 105–18.

Twente, Esther E., *Never Too Old: The Aged in Community Life*, San Francisco, CA: Jossey Bass, 1970.

Van Camp, James V., "Modification of Adult Aggressive Behavior by Using Modeling Films," Ph.D. dissertation, Pasadena, CA: Fuller Theological Seminary Graduate School of Psychology, 1972.

Vinogradov, V. A. and Skvorsov, L. V., *Information Culture: A Key to Social Development and Improvement of Human Existence*, The Hague: SPB Academic Publishers, 1991.

Vollhardt, Lawrence T., "Psychoneuroimmunology: A Literature Review," *American Journal of Orthopsychiatry* 61 (January 1991), pp. 35–47.

Voloshin, Metro, "The Information Revolution and the Library Community, The Good and Bad," *West Virginia Libraries* 41 (Summer 1988), pp. 10–13.

Warner, Lucy, "The Myth of Bibliotherapy," *School Library Journal* (October 1980), pp. 107–11.

Williams, Frederick and Pavlik, John V. (eds), *The People's Right to Know: Media, Democracy and the Information Highway*, Hillsdale, NJ: L. Erlbaum Associates, 1993.

Wolf, Fredric M. *et al.*, "A Controlled Experiment in Teaching Students to Respond to Patients' Emotional Concerns," *Journal of Medical Education* 62 (January 1987), pp. 25–34.

Yager, Edwin K., "Subliminal Therapy: Utilizing the Unconscious Mind," *Medical Hypnoanalysis Journal* 2 (December 1987), pp. 138–47.

Zachariae, R. *et al.*, "Effect of Psychological Intervention in the Form of Relaxation and Guided Imagery on Cellular Immune Function in Normal Healthy Subjects: An Overview," *Psychother. Psychosom.* 54 (1990), pp. 32–39.

Index